Fecal Incontinence and Constipation in Children

Case Studies

Fecal Incontinence and Constipation in Children

Case Studies

Edited by

Onnalisa Nash, MS, CPNP
Center for Colorectal and Pelvic Reconstruction Surgery
Nationwide Children's Hospital
Columbus, Ohio, USA

Julie M. Choueiki, MSN, RN, CPEN
Center for Colorectal and Pelvic Reconstruction Surgery
Nationwide Children's Hospital
Columbus, Ohio, USA

Marc A. Levitt, MD
Center for Colorectal and Pelvic Reconstruction Surgery
Nationwide Children's Hospital
The Ohio State University
Columbus, Ohio, USA

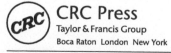

CRC Press
Taylor & Francis Group
Boca Raton London New York

CRC Press is an imprint of the
Taylor & Francis Group, an **informa** business

CRC Press
Taylor & Francis Group
6000 Broken Sound Parkway NW, Suite 300
Boca Raton, FL 33487-2742

© 2020 by Taylor & Francis Group, LLC
CRC Press is an imprint of Taylor & Francis Group, an Informa business

No claim to original U.S. Government works

Printed on acid-free paper

International Standard Book Number-13: 978-0-367-15161-4 (Paperback)
978-0-367-15180-5 (Hardback)

Visit the Taylor & Francis Web site at
http://www.taylorandfrancis.com

and the CRC Press Web site at
http://www.crcpress.com

Contents

Preface

Patients with anorectal malformations (ARMs), Hirschsprung disease (HD), fecal incontinence from a variety of conditions, and colonic motility disorders often require care from specialists across a variety of fields throughout their lives. These include colorectal surgery, urology, gynecology, and GI motility, as well as orthopedics, neurosurgery, anesthesia, pathology, radiology, psychology, social work, and nutrition, amongst many others. Perhaps most important to their achievement of a good functional result is their connection to superb nursing care.

Having met many parents with newborns diagnosed with colorectal problems, I have made several observations. First, no parent ever thinks their child could have a problem with stooling—this is a physiologic ability that is taken for granted. When told this is a problem, they are usually shocked. Second, when discussing with parents that their child will need surgery to correct their colorectal anatomy, they do not focus on the surgical technique and elegance of the anal reconstruction, as I do. Instead, they focus on whether that technique will allow their child to stool without difficulty, and whether school, sleep overs, and overnight camp will be options for them. As surgeons, we need to remember this—we always need to understand what it is that the family wishes for us to deliver to them. As proud of our surgical skills as we are, it is the functional outcome that matters most to our patients.

I like to say that a complex colorectal operation takes about 4 hours to perform, but in order to get a good result, it takes an additional 96 hours of work—the vast majority of which involves nursing care. From the very beginning of my journey in the field of pediatric colorectal surgery, which began in 1992 as a budding medical student, the value of a good nursing partner became clear to me. Patients and their families tell nurses things they would never tell their doctors. Nurses have a spirit about them that is unique—the genuine devotion to helping their patient and never seeming to want anything in return other than the patient's smile. Their skills in identifying problems, solving them, being willing to get down in the weeds, and always striving to fill the gaps are unique to the profession.

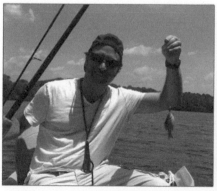 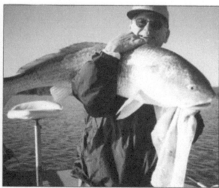

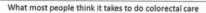

| What most people think it takes to do colorectal care | What it actually takes to do colorectal care |

We have attempted in this book to capture some of these special moments represented in the illustrated cases you are about to encounter. We strove to help other caregivers understand the daily struggle of improving a patient's quality of life and to convey to the readers of this book the skills and tricks to achieve good results. I am so convinced, and often shout from the rooftops that, without my nursing partners, I would have achieved very little as a surgeon. It was an honor

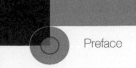

to work on this book with them and to have my name appear as an author beside theirs. We hope you enjoy reading this book and that it helps you help many children. If we have achieved that lofty goal, then we will feel very gratified.

I am forever indebted to the model of education my father, a neurologist, taught me using cases to illustrate learning points, which were codified originally in his books *Neurology for the House Officer* and *Case Studies in Neurology for the House Officer*. Both of my parents, Eva and Larry Levitt, helped me to learn empathy and the importance of hard work. I also wish to thank Shary, my wife, and my children, Sam, Raquel, and Jess who generously gave me up so I could spend time helping patients; their confidence in me and tireless support are the basis of my success.

Marc A. Levitt, MD

Note: Case studies in this book are derived from actual patients. Identifying information such as gender or age may have been altered.

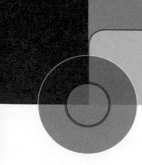

Contributors

Cheryl Baxter, MSN, CPNP
Center for Colorectal and Pelvic Reconstruction Surgery
Nationwide Children's Hospital
Columbus, Ohio

Kristina Booth, MSN, FNP
Center for Colorectal and Pelvic Reconstruction Surgery
Nationwide Children's Hospital
Columbus, Ohio

Julie M. Choueiki, MSN, RN, CPEN
Center for Colorectal and Pelvic Reconstruction Surgery
Nationwide Children's Hospital
Columbus, Ohio

Sara Cramer, BSN, RN
Center for Colorectal and Pelvic Reconstruction Surgery
Nationwide Children's Hospital
Columbus, Ohio

Cassie do Carmo, BSN, RN
Center for Colorectal and Pelvic Reconstruction Surgery
Nationwide Children's Hospital
Columbus, Ohio

Stephanie Dolan, MSN, NP
Division of Colorectal Surgery
The Ohio State University Wexner Medical Center
Columbus, Ohio

Sarah Driesbach, MSN, FNP
Center for Colorectal and Pelvic Reconstruction Surgery
Nationwide Children's Hospital
Columbus, Ohio

Alicia Finn, APRN
Division of Colorectal Surgery
The Ohio State University Wexner Medical Center
Columbus, Ohio

Meghan Fisher, BSN, RN
Center for Colorectal and Pelvic Reconstruction Surgery
Nationwide Children's Hospital
Columbus, Ohio

Alessandra Gasior, DO
Center for Colorectal and Pelvic Reconstruction
    Surgery
Nationwide Children's Hospital
and
Division of Colorectal Surgery
The Ohio State University Wexner Medical Center
Columbus, Ohio

Julie Gerberick, MS, RN, CEN
Center for Colorectal and Pelvic Reconstruction
    Surgery
Nationwide Children's Hospital
Columbus, Ohio

Katrina Hall, MA, CCLS
Center for Colorectal and Pelvic Reconstruction Surgery
Nationwide Children's Hospital
Columbus, Ohio

Charae Keys, MSW, LISW-S
Center for Colorectal and Pelvic Reconstruction Surgery
Nationwide Children's Hospital
Columbus, Ohio

Scott Lake, APRN
Division of Colorectal Surgery
The Ohio State University Wexner Medical Center
Columbus, Ohio

Stacie Leeper, MSN, CPNP
Center for Colorectal and Pelvic Reconstruction Surgery
Nationwide Children's Hospital
Columbus, Ohio

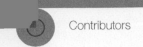

Marc A. Levitt, MD
Center for Colorectal and Pelvic Reconstruction Surgery
Nationwide Children's Hospital
and
The Ohio State University
Columbus, Ohio

Leah Moore, BSN, RN
Center for Colorectal and Pelvic Reconstruction Surgery
Nationwide Children's Hospital
Columbus, Ohio

Onnalisa Nash, MS, CPNP
Center for Colorectal and Pelvic Reconstruction Surgery
Nationwide Children's Hospital
Columbus, Ohio

Lindsay Reilly, MSN, FNP
Center for Colorectal and Pelvic Reconstruction Surgery
Nationwide Children's Hospital
Columbus, Ohio

Natalie Rose, BSN, RN
Center for Colorectal and Pelvic Reconstruction Surgery
Nationwide Children's Hospital
Columbus, Ohio

Rose Lucey Schroedl, PhD
Center for Colorectal and Pelvic Reconstruction Surgery
Nationwide Children's Hospital
Columbus, Ohio

Erin M. Shann, BSN, RN
Center for Colorectal and Pelvic Reconstruction Surgery
Nationwide Children's Hospital
Columbus, Ohio

Amber Traugott, MD
Division of Colorectal Surgery
The Ohio State University Wexner Medical Center
Columbus, Ohio

Catherine Trimble, MSN, FNP
Center for Colorectal and Pelvic Reconstruction Surgery
Nationwide Children's Hospital
Columbus, Ohio

Stephanie J. Vyrostek, BSN, RN
Center for Colorectal and Pelvic Reconstruction Surgery
Nationwide Children's Hospital
Columbus, Ohio

Andrea Wagner, MSN, CPNP
Center for Colorectal and Pelvic Reconstruction Surgery
Nationwide Children's Hospital
Columbus, Ohio

Laura J. Weaver, MA
Center for Colorectal and Pelvic Reconstruction Surgery
Nationwide Children's Hospital
Columbus, Ohio

Pooja Zahora, MSN, FNP
Center for Colorectal and Pelvic Reconstruction Surgery
Nationwide Children's Hospital
Columbus, Ohio

Julie Zipfel, BSN, RN
Center for Colorectal and Pelvic Reconstruction Surgery
Nationwide Children's Hospital
Columbus, Ohio

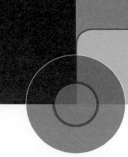

Acknowledgments

We are grateful to the colleagues listed below for the support they provide in the care of patients, their individual roles in our wonderful and collaborative team, and their help in organizing various aspects of this book.

- Katrina Abram
- Brent Adler
- Hira Ahmad
- Neetu Bali
- Jillean Bastian
- Morris Brown
- Christina Ching
- Marissa Condon
- Jackie Cronau
- Daniel DaJusta
- Katherine Deans
- Karen Diefenbach
- Carlo DiLorenzo
- Rob Dyckes
- Pam Edson
- Adrienne Flood
- Molly Fuchs
- Devin Halleran
- Geri Hewitt
- Libbey Hoang
- Jennie Hoffman
- Ronda Hutt
- Venkata R. Jayanthi
- Victoria Lane
- Jeffrey Leonard
- Vickie Leonhardt
- Peter Lu
- Carol Maynard
- Kate McCracken
- Connor McDanel
- Emily McDowell
- Lauryn Michaels
- Peter Minnenci
- Dennis Minzler
- Larry Moss
- Erin Ney
- Kim Osborne
- Allison Pegg
- Gil Peri
- Jeb Phillips
- Ron Pontius
- Patrick Queen
- Raquel Quintanilla Amoros
- Carlos Reck
- Brenda Ruth
- Danielle Sabol
- Steve Sales
- Stephanie Savko
- Alicia Shoemaker
- Tori Smart
- Seryna Smith
- Rachael Subleski
- Benjamin Thompson
- Mandy Thompson
- Casey Thurston
- Bethanne Tilson
- Kathleen Tucker
- Karla Vaz
- Alejandra Vilanova Sanchez
- Jody Wall
- Renee Wells Carpenter
- Kara Wheeler
- Erin Willet
- Kent Williams
- Richard Wood
- Desalegn Yacob

PART

I

BOWEL MANAGEMENT

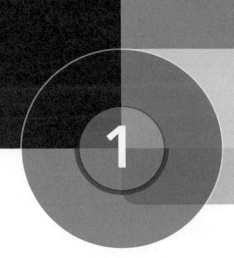

General guidelines for bowel management

STEPHANIE J. VYROSTEK

Bowel management is an outpatient program used to treat fecal incontinence. The clinician selects an appropriate treatment modality, either oral stimulant laxatives or a mechanical program (once daily rectal or antegrade enema). The therapy is adjusted throughout the course of a devoted week according to the patient report and daily abdominal radiograph findings. Whether using an oral stimulant laxative or rectal enema washout, the goal of treatment in both cases is to stimulate a daily bowel movement and empty the colon. The child should then not have another bowel movement or soiling for 24 hours until the next treatment and thereby will be clean and able to wear normal underwear.

The week begins with a contrast enema. This image provides information regarding the shape and size of the colon. Additionally, the speed at which a child evacuates contrast, as seen on subsequent abdominal radiographs, can provide valuable information from which one can infer the colonic motility. The contrast also cleans the colon of residual stool, giving the patient an empty colon to start the week of treatment. If after a contrast enema the patient still has a significant fecal burden, an at home bowel clean out is given prior to starting a mechanical program or laxative trial. The colon must be radiographically clean before starting either program.

TREATMENT MODALITY: MECHANICAL PROGRAM OR STIMULANT LAXATIVES?

The clinician should consider whether the patient has good or poor potential for bowel control when selecting the treatment modality for the bowel management week. Patients with a good potential for bowel control typically respond very well to a stimulant laxative and water-soluble fiber therapies, but may benefit from rectal or antegrade enemas for a period of time depending on if there is dilation of the rectum and rectosigmoid that may impair rectal sensation or if they have never learned to have bowel control. They also become clean quickly and enjoy being clean, which sets them up for success when they try future laxative therapy. Patients with poor potential for bowel control benefit from a mechanical program (rectal or antegrade enema). Each regimen must be tailored to the needs of the patient, with particular attention paid to the age of the child, the underlying diagnosis (e.g., anorectal malformation, Hirschsprung disease, functional constipation, spinal conditions, sacrococcygeal teratoma), and the child's "potential" for bowel control (i.e., their inherent ability to have voluntary bowel movements).

POTENTIAL FOR BOWEL CONTROL

There are multiple factors that can be used to assess whether a patient has good potential for bowel control. These include maturity and a commitment to potty train, anal anatomy, anal sphincters, normal sacral anatomy, normal spinal anatomy (and thus normal innervation of the anorectum), and an anoplasty (surgically created anus) located in the center of the sphincter mechanism *and* without stricture or prolapse. We will review these six factors and how each can affect children with an anorectal malformation (ARM), Hirschsprung disease (HD), functional constipation, and spinal processes (see Figure 1.1).

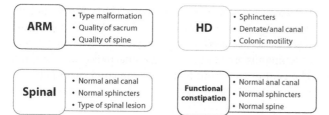

Figure 1.1 Predictors of continence. ARM = anorectal malformation, HD = Hirschsprung disease.

MATURITY AND COMMITMENT TO POTTY TRAINING

The age at which children begin potty training is different in a variety of countries and cultures. There are certain parts of the world that require the child to be potty trained to go to organized schooling such as preschool. This leads to increasing pressure on the parents to get their children in normal underwear as early as possible. Developmental delay also plays a significant role in whether a child is able to potty train when it is socially expected. Children with ARM, HD, functional constipation, and spinal processes will struggle with these societal "norms" as they try to potty train.

ANAL ANATOMY

The anal canal and dentate line are vital for differentiating between solid stool, liquid stool, and gas. If there is damage to the anal canal, the child will be unsuccessful in recognizing the difference between the three and being able to pass them when socially acceptable. This could lead to stooling accidents.

i. Children with an anorectal malformation almost always lack a dentate line and normal anal canal as those failed to develop while in utero. These patients require a surgically created anal canal.

ii. Those with Hirschsprung disease should have an intact dentate line when born; however, this can be damaged by the surgical dissection during a pull-through surgery.

iii. Children with functional constipation have a normal anal canal and dentate line, and those with spinal anomalies typically have a normal anal canal and dentate line, but, with the effect of poor nerve innervation, they may not function properly.

ANAL SPHINCTERS

Intact sphincters are required for a child to have the ability to squeeze their anus; this includes both voluntary (skeletal) and involuntary (smooth) muscles. The anal sphincters may be relatively normal in children with an anorectal malformation who have a low malformation (perineal fistula, rectobulbar fistula, vestibular fistula, and short common channel cloaca), and slightly underdeveloped in those children with higher malformations (rectoprostatic fistula, bladder neck fistula, and long common channel cloaca). The quality of the sphincter in Hirschsprung disease is very good, but may have hypertonic smooth muscle that does not allow relaxation (absent RAIR—rectoanal inhibitory reflex) and permit stool to pass easily. Anal sphincters that are loose or overstretched in this patient population are typically of an iatrogenic cause. Children with functional constipation have normal anal sphincters, but can have overactive smooth muscles as well, which do not allow them to relax fully while attempting a bowel movement. In children with spinal anomalies, as with the anal canal, the anatomy is normal but the nerve innervation has been interrupted by their spinal anomaly. Disruption of anal sphincters can also be seen in patients who have suffered from pelvic trauma.

SACRAL ANATOMY

The development of the sacrum seems to correlate with the development of the muscles and nerves in the pelvic floor. The underdevelopment of the sacrum typically is only associated with those children with anorectal malformations. In ARM patients, the quality of the sacrum, and therefore the muscles and nerves, can be assessed by calculating the sacral ratio (see Figure 1.2). A ratio greater than 0.7 is considered normal. One below 0.4 is quite hypodeveloped.

SPINAL ANATOMY

The most frequent spinal anomalies treated with a bowel management program are spina bifida, tethered cord, occult spinal dysraphism, myelomeningocele, and sacrococcygeal teratomas. Spinal anomalies can be seen across all patients with ARM, HD, and functional constipation.

ANOPLASTY

A surgically created anus in patients with anorectal malformations has to be placed within the center of the

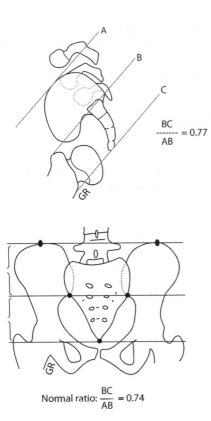

Normal ratio: $\dfrac{BC}{AB} = 0.74$

Figure 1.2 Calculating a sacral ratio.

sphincter complex. This gives the child the best potential for continence as they grow. Even placement slightly out of the center can cause stooling accidents in patients who have the best potential. If there is a stricture or prolapse, this can interfere with successful continence and may need repair prior to potty training.

PROGRAM DETAILS: ENEMAS AND LAXATIVES

ENEMAS

A normal saline enema regimen (usually 15–20 mL/kg) is prescribed to the patient. Glycerin or a gentle soap are first-line stimulants to be added to the saline. Some children may require stronger stimulants such as bisacodyl, but should be maxed out on glycerin and soap prior to trying that medication. Children or their caregivers are instructed to administer the enema slowly over 5–10 minutes, hold the solution in for 5–10 minutes (if given rectally), and sit on the

toilet to evacuate stool for 30 minutes. The type of stimulant, volume, and concentration are adjusted daily during the week as needed according to the patient's tolerance, report of symptoms or soiling, and abdominal radiograph findings. The goal of treatment is to keep the child clean between enemas. See Table 1.1 for standard dosing and titration of saline, glycerin, Castile soap, and bisacodyl.

Table 1.1 Enema formulation

Saline base (rectal or antegrade)
- Volume determined by provider based on contrast study
- 20–30 mL/kg

Glycerin enema (rectal or antegrade)
- Use with saline base
- Glycerin ordered in 5–10 mL increments
- Once 40 mL has been reached, consider adding additional stimulant
- If patient is symptomatic using this (e.g. vomiting/severe abdominal cramping), consider changing stimulant or substitute with Castile soap

X-ray shows:
(a) *No stool burden*:
- Accidents: Decrease glycerin 10 mL
- No accidents: Keep glycerin the same and continue to monitor
(b) *Mild stool burden*:
- Accidents: Increase glycerin 10 mL
- No accidents: Keep glycerin the same and continue to monitor
(c) *Moderate stool burden*:
- Accidents/no accidents: Increase glycerin 10 mL
(d) *Severe stool burden*:
- Accidents/no accidents: Increase glycerin 10 mL

Castile soap enema (rectal or antegrade) use with saline base
- Castile soap ordered in 9 mL increments
- Once 36 mL has been reached, consider adding additional stimulant
- If patient is symptomatic using this (e.g. vomiting/severe abdominal cramping), consider changing stimulant or substitute with baby soap

X-ray shows:
(a) *No stool burden*:
- Accidents: Decrease Castile soap 9 mL
- No accidents: Keep Castile soap the same and continue to monitor
(b) *Mild stool burden*:
- Accidents: Increase Castile soap 9 mL
- No accidents: Keep Castile soap the same and continue to monitor

(Continued)

Table 1.1 (Continued) Enema formulation

(c) *Moderate stool burden*:
- Accidents/no accidents: Increase Castile soap 9 mL

(d) *Severe stool burden*:
- Accidents/no accidents: Increase Castile soap 9 mL

Bisacodyl enema (rectal or antegrade)
- Bisacodyl 10 mg/30 mL
- Ordered in increments of 2.5 mg (7.5 mL)
- Once 30 mg (90 mL) has been reached, consider adding additional stimulant
- If patient is symptomatic using this (e.g. vomiting/severe abdominal cramping) consider changing stimulant

X-ray shows:

(a) *No stool burden*:
- Accidents: Decrease bisacodyl 2.5 mg (7.5 mL)
- No accidents: Keep bisacodyl the same and continue to monitor

(b) *Mild stool burden*:
- Accidents: Increase bisacodyl 5 mg (15 mL)
- No accidents: Keep bisacodyl the same and continue to monitor

(c) Moderate stool burden:
- Accidents/no accidents: Increase bisacodyl 5 mg (15 mL)

(d) *Severe stool burden*:
- Accidents/no accidents: Increase bisacodyl 5 mg (15 mL)

Table 1.2 Laxative protocol and fiber supplements

Senna laxative protocol — after APN or MD assesses and classifies stool burden on X-ray
- Senna ordered in 7.5 mg, 15 mg, or 25 mg increments
- Max dose dependent on patient's tolerance
- Used in conjunction with water-soluble fiber

X-ray shows:

(a) *No stool burden*:
- Accidents: Decrease laxative by half a tab or square (7.5 mg or 12.5 mg depending on dose)
- No accidents: Keep laxative the same and continue to monitor

(b) *Mild stool burden*:
- Accidents: Keep laxative the same and consider increasing water-soluble fiber
- No accidents: Keep laxative the same and continue to monitor

(c) *Moderate stool burden*:
- Accidents/no accidents: Increase laxative by a tab or square (15 mg or 25 mg depending on dose)

(d) *Severe stool burden*:
- Accidents/no accidents: Give rectal sodium phosphate enema (OTC, pediatric for children <2yo, adult for >2yo) AND increase laxative by tab or square (15 mg or 25 mg depending on dose)

Water-soluble fiber protocol—after APN or MD assesses and classifies stool burden on X-ray
- Water-soluble fiber ordered in 2 g increments
- Max dose dependent on patient's tolerance
- Used alone or in conjunction with senna or loperamide

X-ray shows:

(a) *No stool burden*:
- Loose stool and/or accidents: Increase water-soluble fiber 2 g
- No accidents: Keep water-soluble fiber the same and continue to monitor

(b) *Mild stool burden*:
- Loose stool and/or accidents: Increase water-soluble fiber 2 g
- No accidents: Keep water-soluble fiber the same and continue to monitor

(c) *Moderate stool burden*:
- Loose stool and/or accidents: Increase water-soluble fiber 2 g
- No accidents: Keep water-soluble fiber the same and continue to monitor

(d) *Severe stool burden*:
- Accidents/no accidents: Give rectal sodium phosphate enema (OTC, pediatric for children <2yo, adult for >2yo) AND decrease water-soluble fiber by 2 g

LAXATIVES

Senna-based oral stimulant laxatives are the first choice for treatment based on their ability to provoke the colon to contract and empty the stool burden. Stool softeners or osmotic laxatives (e.g. polyethylene glycol) should be avoided because they make the stool soft, but do not provoke stool to empty. The laxative dose is determined from interpretation of the contrast enema, age and weight of the patient, and previously tried regimens. The patient is observed for 24 hours after laxative administration. If the child does not stool within 24 hours, their caregivers are instructed to administer an over the counter rectal enema to evacuate rectal stool burden. After the enema, the laxative dose is increased. In contrast, if the patient stools multiple times and the abdominal radiograph does not have a significant stool burden, the laxative dose can be decreased. Water-soluble fiber is prescribed in conjunction with laxatives to add bulk to the stool and to decrease the occurrence of watery stools. The laxative and fiber dosages are adjusted daily during the week as needed according to the patient's tolerance, report of symptoms or soiling, and abdominal radiograph findings. The goal of treatment is one to two formed bowel movements per day and no soiling accidents. See Table 1.2 for standard dosing and titration of senna and water-soluble fiber supplementation.

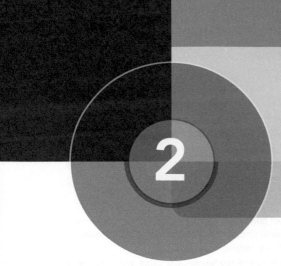

Bowel management program setup: The basics and long-term follow-up

STEPHANIE J. VYROSTEK
AND LAURA J. WEAVER

The creation and maintenance of a successful bowel management program (BMP) is an ongoing and evolving endeavor. Such a program consistently presents new challenges to overcome, which allows for institutional growth and development of the program. Some key drivers to identify prior to signing up patients should include:

- Time frame (e.g., one-week program, monthly)
- Number of patients and anticipated family participation
- Institutional accommodations
- Long-term follow-up

We will discuss each point and provide recommendations for a successful program.

TIME FRAME

Bowel management programs should include direct communication with patients and families for a minimum of 1 week. This time frame allows the provider caring for that patient to review applicable studies at the first meeting and troubleshoot any circumstances during the week to help the child achieve social continence. The provider may choose to see the child in clinic multiple times or to have email or phone communication throughout this 7-day period.

A typical week may look like this (Figure 2.1):

NUMBER OF PATIENTS

The amount of nursing support is vital, as nurses are the ones triaging all family inquiries. It is imperative not to schedule too many patients, as spreading the nurse too thin can cause less individual attention to the bowel management participants and cause them to feel unsupported, which could in turn negatively impact their outcomes. Having this direct contact and support network makes the patient and family feel valued. The number of patients a program can handle will need to be discussed with nursing staff and administrators, and constantly re-evaluated to make sure goals are being met in order to help as many children as possible, without overwhelming the staff or infrastructure.

Family participation is vital to the success of the child's bowel management program. The entire family has to be on board and needs to understand the "burden" of this therapy required to achieve success. Families need to be set up for success with realistic expectations for their child's potential for continence. The family reports of how things are going when the child is not in clinic are vital for the providers who use this information, as well as the radiograph images to adjust medications. The data provided must be detailed and allow your team to know exactly what has happened at home during the

Day 1	Day 2	Day 3	Day 4	Day 5	Day 6	Day 7
• Contrast enema • Clinic visit	• X-ray • Patient report	• X-ray • Patient report	• X-ray • Clinic visit	• X-ray • Patient report	• X-ray • Patient report	• X-ray • Clinic visit

Figure 2.1 Typical week of bowel management.

Daily enema program chart

	1st Thursday	Friday
Normal saline amount (mL)		
Glycerin amount (mL)		
Castile soap amount (mL)		
Other medicines (name and dose)		
Diet instructions		
Time enema started		
Time enema finished		
How long enema took to go in (minutes)		
How long enema stayed in (minutes)		
Any symptoms when giving enema?		
Total time seated on the toilet (minutes)		
Accidents: How many? Time? Description?		

Figure 2.2 Enema program report sheet.

individualized program. See Figures 2.2 through 2.4 for examples of family report sheets for the enema program and the laxative programs.

INSTITUTIONAL ACCOMMODATIONS

A bowel management program will likely bring an increase of patients to a clinic, and this will also affect the institution as a whole. These patients will impact radiology (ultrasound, magnetic resonance imaging [MRI], interventional radiology), pharmacy, urology, gynecology, gastroenterology and neurosurgery, as well as the operating room. Including each team in the discussion of flow and impact is essential to success and each department has their own part to play in the success of the program. Having the support of the institution and all the other departments will help the patients feel valued across the organization. Preliminary meetings with all involved parties is a key step in the process.

Daily medicine program for hypermotility chart

	1st Thursday	Friday
Kind and amount of medicine		
Time medicine given		
Kind and amount of fiber		
Diet instructions		
Voluntary bowel movements: Amount and description		
Accidents/soiling: Time, amount and description		

Figure 2.3 Medicine program for hypermotility.

Daily medicine program for hypomotility chart

	1st Thursday	Friday
Kind and amount of laxative		
Time laxative given		
Kind and amount of fiber		
Other medicines (name and dose)		
Diet instructions		
Voluntary bowel movements: Amount and description		
Accidents/soiling: Time, amount and description		

Figure 2.4 Medicine program for hypomotility.

LONG-TERM FOLLOW-UP

When the week-long program has finished, there is still ongoing management that must be maintained. Losing sight of the long-term efforts that need to go into this patient population is a recipe for poor outcomes.

Initially, close follow-up is required to confirm that the patient's regimen is continuing to work and all concerns the family may be facing upon returning home can be addressed. This is routinely done at 1 month and 3 months, after the completion of the bowel management program. The goal would be then to move to annual follow-up until any future intervention is needed.

In the authors' center, the provider completes the follow-up intervals at 1 month and 3 months in clinic or over the phone and the annual follow-up in person in clinic. Prior to each follow-up appointment, the patient gets an abdominal X-ray. They also complete a questionnaire about their regimen and certain pertinent continent and quality of life scores. The scores currently used are the Baylor Social Continence Scale, Cleveland Clinic Constipation Scoring System, and Vancouver Dysfunctional Elimination Syndrome Survey with the addition of Pediatric Quality of Life at the annual visits (Figure 2.5). The provider reviews the X-ray image and the outcomes of the patient's scores and then conducts the clinic visit or the phone interview with the family. If at any time the provider feels the need to adjust the follow-up schedule, it is done while still collecting the completed scores at the predetermined intervals (Figure 2.6).

The Baylor Social Continence Scale, Cleveland Clinic Constipation Scoring System, Vancouver Dysfunctional Elimination Syndrome Survey, and Pediatric Quality of Life are also collected prior to the patient completing the bowel management program. This provides the opportunity to see the patient's objective progress, as well as areas for growth. See Figure 2.7 for an example of a bowel management flowsheet for follow-up care.

Urinary questions — Asked by the provider
- Any changes to your child's urinary status?
- Any UTI or UTI symptoms?

Stooling questions — Asked by the provider and assessed on abdominal X-ray
- How many bowel movements per day?
- Are they accidents or voluntary?
- What time of day do they occur?

Regimen questions — Assessed and changed by the provider
- What is the current regimen your child is on?
- Is your child tolerating that regimen?
- Are there any barriers you have experienced since being home?

Figure 2.5 Example question for follow up.

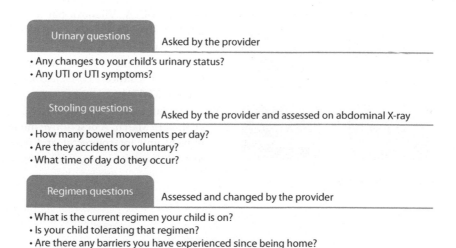

Intake (virtual option)	1 month (virtual option)	3 month (virtual option)	1 year
• Baylor	• Baylor	• Baylor	• Baylor
• Cleveland	• Cleveland	• Cleveland	• Cleveland
• Vancouver	• Vancouver	• Vancouver	• Vancouver
• Peds QL			• Peds QL

Figure 2.6 Survey collection intervals.

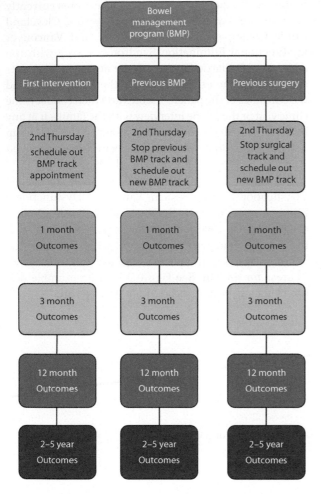

Figure 2.7 Bowel management flowsheet for follow-up care.

SUGGESTED READINGS

Afshar, K., Mirbagheri, A., Scott, H., & MacNeily, A. E. 2009 October. Development of a symptom score for dysfunctional elimination syndrome. *Journal of Urology,* 182(4 Suppl), 1939–1943.

Agachan, F., Chen, T., Pfeifer, J., Reissman, P., & Wexner, S. D. 1996 June. A constipation scoring system to simplify evaluation and management of constipated patients. *Diseases of the Colon Rectum,* 39(6), 681–685.

Bischoff, A., & Levitt, M. 2009. Treatment of fecal incontinence with a comprehensive bowel management program. *Journal of Pediatric Surgery,* 44, 1278–1284.

Brandt, M. L., Daigneau, C., Graviss, E. A., Naik-Mathuria, B., Fitch, M. E., & Washburn, K. K. 2007 June. Validation of the Baylor Continence Scale in children with anorectal malformations. *Journal of Pediatric Surgery,* 42(6), 1015–1021; discussion 1021.

Levitt, M. A., & Pena, A. 2010. Pediatric fecal incontinence: A surgeon's perspective. *Pediatrics in Review,* 31, 91–98.

Reck-Burneo, C. A., Vilanova-Sanchez, A., Gasior, A. et al. 2018. A structured bowel management program for patients with severe functional constipation can help decrease emergency department visits, hospital admissions, and healthcare costs. *Journal of Pediatric Surgery,* 53(9), 1737–1741.

Vilanova-Sanchez, A., Halleran, D. R., Reck-Burneo, C. A. et al. 2019 March. A descriptive model for a multidisciplinary unit for colorectal and pelvic malformation. *Journal Pediatric Surgery,* 54(3), 479–485.

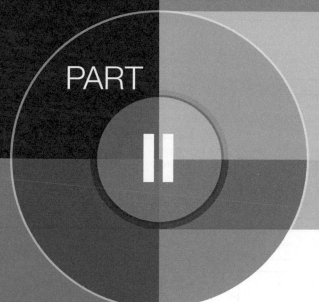

PART II

ANORECTAL MALFORMATIONS

INTRODUCTION

Onnalisa Nash

Anorectal malformation (ARM) describes the congenital problem of an absent anal opening or one that is in the wrong place. These anomalies are a spectrum of disorders involving the distal anus, rectum, and frequently the urinary and gynecologic system. The prevalence is about 1 in 5000 births worldwide. After surgical repair, patients frequently require treatment for constipation and/or fecal incontinence.

Fecal and urinary incontinence can occur even with an excellent anatomic repair usually related to associated spinal or pelvic hypo or abnormal development. An effective bowel management program is the most beneficial way to improve the quality of life of a patient with these concerns.

The most frequent morbidity encountered after surgical repair of an ARM is constipation. It is also the most important problem to avoid after definitive repair, starting right after repair or after colostomy closure as the case may be. If constipation is not avoided and well treated postoperatively, an enlarged rectum and sigmoid can result, which can lead to fecal impaction and overflow incontinence.

Less frequent than constipation, some patients experience soiling. In a patient with a good prognosis, this may manifest as overflow incontinence (meaning the patient has the potential for bowel control but soils due to regular impactions). It may also represent true fecal incontinence (meaning the patient lacks the ability to have a voluntary bowel movement) in cases of very high malformations, and when there is an associated spinal abnormality and/or an abnormal sacrum. A contrast enema along with the sacral ratio and spinal imaging is helpful in discerning this information. The ARM Index (Figure II.1) is helpful in predicting continence in patients with ARM.

ARM INDEX

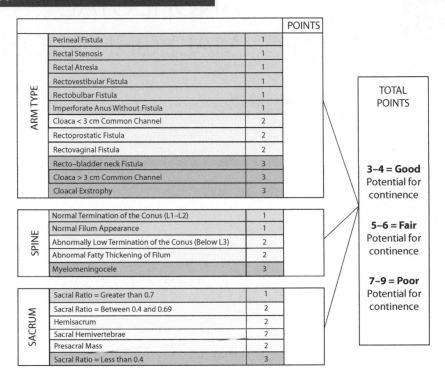

		POINTS
ARM TYPE	Perineal Fistula	1
	Rectal Stenosis	1
	Rectal Atresia	1
	Rectovestibular Fistula	1
	Rectobulbar Fistula	1
	Imperforate Anus Without Fistula	1
	Cloaca < 3 cm Common Channel	2
	Rectoprostatic Fistula	2
	Rectovaginal Fistula	2
	Recto–bladder neck Fistula	3
	Cloaca > 3 cm Common Channel	3
	Cloacal Exstrophy	3
SPINE	Normal Termination of the Conus (L1–L2)	1
	Normal Filum Appearance	1
	Abnormally Low Termination of the Conus (Below L3)	2
	Abnormal Fatty Thickening of Filum	2
	Myelomeningocele	3
SACRUM	Sacral Ratio = Greater than 0.7	1
	Sacral Ratio = Between 0.4 and 0.69	2
	Hemisacrum	2
	Sacral Hemivertebrae	2
	Presacral Mass	2
	Sacral Ratio = Less than 0.4	3

TOTAL POINTS

3–4 = Good
Potential for continence

5–6 = Fair
Potential for continence

7–9 = Poor
Potential for continence

Figure II.1 **(See color insert.)** Arm Index.

The ARM Index shown has a "report card" format that can help predict continence potential in a patient with ARM. The three areas that are assessed are the type of malformation, the quality of the spine, and the quality of the sacrum. Using the ARM Index report card, points are given in each area, which are then added to determine the score for each patient. The patients with good potential for continence will have a score of 3–4, fair potential for continence will have a score of 5–6, and poor potential will have a score of 7–9.

Once the ARM index score is determined, the prognosis for continence can be predicted. If a patient's ARM Index indicates good potential for continence, the practitioner and family can plan for the probability of success with a laxative regimen. If a patient's diagnosis points to a poor prognosis, the practitioner and parents should plan for the likelihood that that child will need a mechanical bowel regimen to remain clean. Patients with fair potential usually need to be started on a mechanical regimen at first, but may be able to transition to a medical regimen (laxatives) as they grow older. As the child matures, the likelihood of achieving bowel control generally improves.

The cases we will consider in this section include:

- A patient with good surgical anatomy with good potential for bowel control
- A patient with good surgical anatomy with fair potential for bowel control
- A patient with good surgical anatomy with poor potential for bowel control
- A patient in need of bowel management with the need for urologic reconstruction
- A young adult with prior surgery for ARM, with fecal incontinence
- A patient with ARM who is a sacral nerve stimulator candidate

SUGGESTED READINGS

Lane, V., Wood, R., Reck, C., & Levitt, M. 2017. Pediatric Colorectal and Pelvic Surgery: Case Studies. CRC Press.

Wood, R., & Levitt, M. 2018. Anorectal malformations. *Clinics in Colon and Rectal Surgery*. 31(02), 061–070.

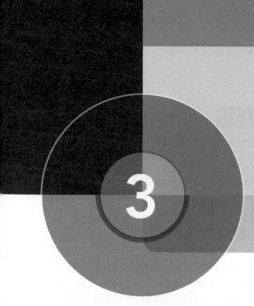
A patient with good surgical anatomy after an anorectal malformation (ARM) repair with good potential for bowel control

ERIN M. SHANN

CASE HISTORY

A 6-year-old boy, adopted from China at the age of 3, comes to your clinic. He was born with an anorectal malformation (perineal fistula) that was repaired as a newborn in China as a primary posterior sagittal anorectoplasty (PSARP). He now has daily soiling with his home enema regimen of 400 mL normal saline, 15 mL glycerin, and 10 mL Castile soap. His spine and urological system are normal and his lateral sacral ratio is 0.78 (refer to the figure "ARM Index" in the color insert).

QUESTION 3.1

What is your assessment of his potential for continence?

A. Good
B. Fair
C. Poor

Answer: This patient had a perineal fistula repaired, which is a low malformation. He has no abnormalities with his sacrum and no signs of tethered cord. His sacral ratio is within the normal range, which is greater than 0.7. Based on this information, the patient has a good potential for bowel control (Answer = A).

During the initial evaluation of the patient, physical exam findings were normal (the anoplasty was well placed, without stricture or rectal prolapse), and a contrast study was performed to assess the anatomy. The prior surgery was done well.

A contrast enema was performed and is shown in Figures 3.1 and 3.2.

A post-evacuation film is shown in Figure 3.3.

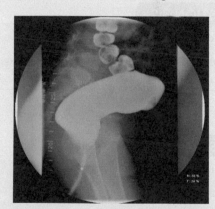

Figure 3.1 Contrast enema, lateral view.

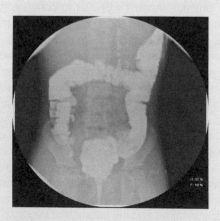

Figure 3.2 Contrast enema, frontal view.

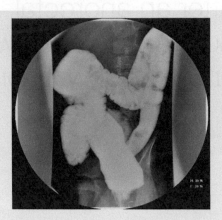

Figure 3.3 Post-evacuation radiograph.

What does the contrast study show?

Answer: The contrast study shows a mildly redundant sigmoid colon and dilated rectum.

QUESTION 3.3

What regimen would you start?

A. Laxatives and fiber
B. Rectal enemas

Answer: Based on his first evaluation, he was kept on rectal enemas (Answer = B) due to consistently having soiling with his current home regimen of 400 mL normal saline, 15 mL glycerin, and 10 mL Castile soap. He was kept on rectal enemas and not switched to a laxative and fiber regimen because he has never been "clean" of stool and his contrast study showed dilation of the rectum.

We changed him to a regimen of 350 mL normal saline, 20 mL glycerin, and 15 mL Castile soap to see if this would help the colon become clean daily and allow him to avoid soiling. The strength of his flush was increased to see if it would provoke a larger bowel movement at enema time. Despite this change, stool accidents occurred approximately 18 hours after the rectal enema was administered and the patient had begun to become resistant to the enema administration.

QUESTION 3.4

What should the next steps be?

A. Stay on rectal enemas
B. Get urology clearance and perform a Malone appendicostomy
C. Start laxatives and fiber
D. Attend a bowel management week

Answer: A Malone appendicostomy was performed (Answer = B) given his age, his persistent soiling, and intolerance of rectal enemas due to him being anally defensive. Despite him having good potential for bowel control, we still felt a mechanical program was best at this point in his life. Once this is achieved, it could be the bridge to future continence using laxatives. Before he was able to have the Malone appendicostomy performed, he needed to receive the "golden ticket" from urology.

The "golden ticket" is when urology determines the appendix is not needed for a Mitrofanoff or any other urological repair. If that were to be the case the urologic procedure and the Malone can be done at the same operation. All of his urology testing was normal and he needed no urological surgery done at the same time as the Malone. At one month postoperatively from the Malone, he attended a bowel management week.

DAY 1

Patient report:

- Regimen: 350 mL normal saline, 20 mL glycerin , and 15 mL Castile soap
- An abdominal X-ray was performed (Figure 3.4)

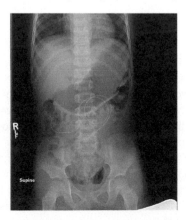

Figure 3.4 Day 1 X-ray.

QUESTION 3.5

What does the X-ray show?

A. The X-ray is clean
B. Small amount of stool throughout the colon
C. Moderate stool in the ascending colon and the rectum
D. Stool only in the rectum

Answer: There is moderate stool in the ascending colon and in the rectum (Answer=C). The colon needs to be cleaner.

QUESTION 3.6

What would be your new recommended regimen?

A. 400 mL normal saline and 20 mL glycerin
B. 400 mL normal saline, 20 mL glycerin, and 9 mL Castile soap
C. 350 mL normal saline, 20 mL glycerin, and 15 mL Castile soap
D. 450 mL normal saline, 20 mL glycerin, and 15 mL Castile soap

Answer: The patient was placed on 450 mL normal saline, 20 mL glycerin, and 15 mL Castile soap (Answer=D). Normal saline was increased to help fill the colon more, thereby helping the colon to empty.

QUESTION 3.7

What does the X-ray show?

A. Stool only in the ascending colon
B. Clean X-ray, no stool
C. Stool in the ascending colon but clean throughout

Answer: The X-ray is very clean now which means the flush is strong. There is a small amount of stool in the ascending colon. There is no stool accumulation in the transverse, descending colon or rectum (Answer=C).

QUESTION 3.8

Would you change the regimen?

A. The flush is just right, no changes
B. Too strong of a flush, decrease the strength of the regimen
C. The flush is not strong enough, increase the strength of the regimen

Answer: It is recommended to decrease the strength of the flush slightly to help avoid accidents that are being provoked by the stronger flush (Answer=B).

DAY 2

Patient report:

- Regimen: 450 mL normal saline, 20 mL glycerin, and 15 mL Castile soap
- One accident at 19 hours after the flush with some leaking (Figure 3.5)

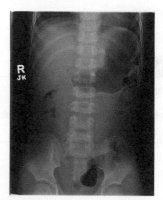

Figure 3.5 Day 2 X-ray.

DAY 3

Patient report:

- Regimen: 400 mL normal saline, 20 mL glycerin, and 9 mL Castile soap
- Family reported an overnight accident

QUESTION 3.9

A new X-ray was obtained. What does it show (Figure 3.6)?

Answer: There is a small amount of stool in the ascending colon which is of no significance. There is still no stool in the transverse, descending colon, or the rectum. This X-ray is again very clean.

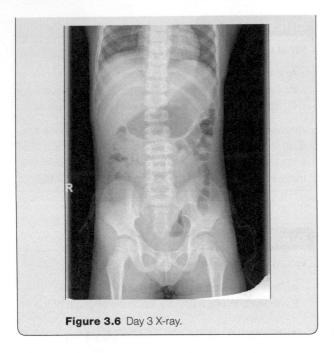

Figure 3.6 Day 3 X-ray.

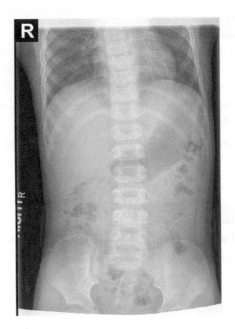

Figure 3.7 Day 4 X-ray, view 1.

QUESTION 3.10

What regimen ingredient would you change?

A. Normal saline
B. Glycerin
C. Castile

Answer: The patient is being overstimulated with the additives glycerin and Castile soap. The patient was taken off of Castile soap because it has a higher stimulation effect on the colon (Answer = C).

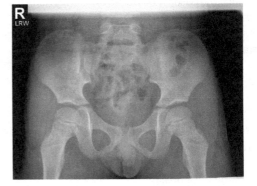

Figure 3.8 Day 4 X-ray, view 2.

DAY 4

Patient report:

- Regimen: 400 mL normal saline and 20 mL glycerin
- Family reported a small overnight accident along with a small daytime accident.
- X-ray shows: Stool in the descending colon and in the rectum (Figures 3.7 and 3.8).

QUESTION 3.11

What does the X-ray show?

Answer: The X-ray now shows stool in the ascending and descending colon, as well as the rectum.

QUESTION 3.12

What would you like to do next?

A. Increase normal saline by 50 mL
B. Decrease glycerin by 10 mL
C. Add fiber to the current regimen
D. Take glycerin out of the regimen

Answer: The patient still needs the additive of the glycerin to help stimulate the colon to provoke a bowel movement. The X-rays have been cleaner, but the patient is still experiencing fecal soiling. Fiber was added to the regimen to help bulk the stool along with keeping the flush of 400 mL normal saline and 20 mL glycerin (Answer = C).

QUESTION 3.14

How would you change the regimen?

A. Keep the regimen the same to give the fiber a chance to help bulk the stool more
B. Take the fiber away, it bulked the stool too much
C. Add 9 mL of Castile soap into the regimen
D. Increase the glycerin by 10 mL

Answer: Glycerin was increased by 10 mL (Answer = D) because the patient was accumulating stool in the descending colon. When a patient is on antegrade flushes or rectal enemas, the goal is to have the descending colon clean of stool.

DAY 5

Patient report:

- Regimen: 400 mL normal saline, and 20 mL glycerin, and 2 g of fiber twice a day
- Family reported an overnight accident and another accident about 22–24 hours after previous flush (Figure 3.9)

DAY 6

Patient report:

- Regimen: 450 mL normal saline, 30 mL glycerin, and 2 g fiber twice a day
- Continues to experience 1–2 episodes of leakage overnight (Figure 3.10)

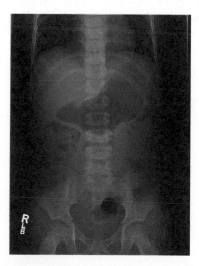

Figure 3.9 Day 5 X-ray.

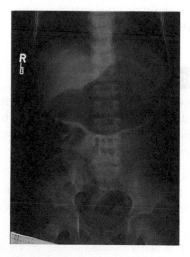

Figure 3.10 Day 6 X-ray.

QUESTION 3.13

What does the X-ray show?

Answer: The X-ray shows stool accumulation in the ascending and descending colon.

QUESTION 3.15

What does the X-ray show?

Answer: The X-ray demonstrates stool accumulation in the rectum.

QUESTION 3.16

It is the last day of bowel management. What will you change the regimen to?

A. Continue same regimen and give the fiber time to bulk the stool
B. Increase the fiber to three times a day
C. Decrease the normal saline, decrease the glycerin, add Castile soap, and take away the fiber

Answer: The regimen for home is 400 mL normal saline, 20 mL glycerin, and 5 mL Castile soap (Answer = C). The fiber was taken away due to stool accumulation on the X-ray. The glycerin was decreased and the Castile soap was added back into the regimen to help provoke more of a bowel movement with the combination of the stimulants.

KEY LEARNING POINTS

1. Malone appendicostomies can be considered for those who are anally defensive to help decrease the psychological component with doing rectal enemas for both the patient and the family.
2. Soiling after the flush with a clean X-ray could mean that the flush is too stimulating and is provoking accidents between flushes.
3. Fiber can be added to the regimen to help bulk the stool to decrease the number of accidents the patient is experiencing.
4. A patient with good potential for bowel control is likely to succeed on a laxative and fiber regimen.
5. If the patient is a good candidate for a laxative and fiber trial, the ultimate decision on when to do this will depend on the family and patient's readiness.

PRESENT DAY

During a phone follow-up appointment, the family reported that the patient was currently doing 400 mL normal saline, 20 mL glycerin, and 9 mL Castile soap via Malone. The patient rarely had accidents, approximately three times per month. The family reported that they occasionally skip a flush over the weekend.

SUGGESTED READING

Reck-Burneo, C. A., Vilanova-Sanchez, A., Gasior, A. C. et al. 2018. A structured bowel management program for patients with severe functional constipation can help decrease emergency department visits, hospital admissions, and health care costs. *Journal of Pediatric Surgery,* 53, 1737–1741.

QUESTION 3.17

Based on how bowel management went and the present day, what would the next steps be for this patient based on their anatomy and their potential for bowel control?

A. Continue same regimen
B. Have patient begin every other day flushes
C. Have patient attend another bowel management week to transition to laxatives

Answer: The family decided to stay on the same daily flush regimen at this time. The family likes the convenience of only having one bowel movement per day. They will consider attending a formal bowel management week for a laxative and fiber trial. Given the patient's good potential for bowel control they would do well on a laxative and fiber trial (Answer = C).

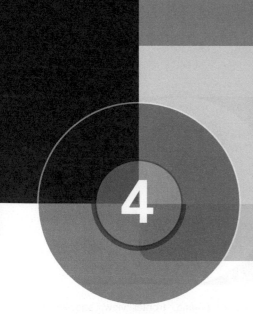

A patient with good surgical anatomy following an anorectal malformation (ARM) repair with fair potential for bowel control

ERIN M. SHANN

CASE HISTORY

A 4-year-old boy comes to your clinic with a history of anorectal malformation (ARM) (rectoprostatic urethral fistula), tethered cord, and sacral dysgenesis, complaining of daily accidents. His initial ARM repair was done at an outside hospital in his first year of life with preceding colostomy as a newborn and subsequent colostomy closure. His current bowel regimen includes lactulose, polyethylene glycol 3350 (MiraLAX), and Fleet enemas to treat constipation.

QUESTION 4.1

What is your assessment of his potential for continence?

A. Need more testing to help determine true potential for continence
B. Good potential for continence

Answer: More testing is needed to determine the true potential for continence (Answer = A).

QUESTION 4.2

What testing would you need?

Answer: A sacral X-ray and a magnetic resonance imaging (MRI) spine are needed to assess his continence potential (Figure 4.1).

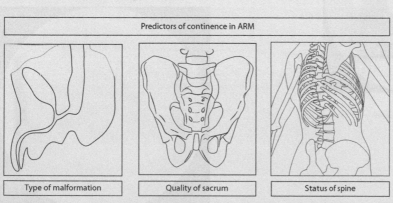

Predictors of continence in ARM

| Type of malformation | Quality of sacrum | Status of spine |

Figure 4.1 Predictors of continence in ARM needed to assess such a patient.

QUESTION 4.3

What are the next steps?

A. Continue current regimen with no additional workup
B. Complete a formal bowel management week with a contrast study
C. Complete a formal bowel management week with a contrast study, renal testing, and an MRI spine
D. Continue current regimen, obtain a contrast study, renal testing, and an MRI spine

Answer: The patient should complete a formal bowel management week, obtain a water soluble contrast study, a renal ultrasound, and a pelvic MRI (Answer = C). A water soluble contrast study is needed to assess the anatomy of the colon to check for redundancy, distention, twists, narrowing, and a widened pre-sacral space (which could indicate a pre-sacral mass). The renal ultrasound is needed to check the health of the kidneys. It is found that most individuals with ARM are prone to have poor kidney health. The pelvic MRI is needed to check for a pre-sacral mass and a remnant of the original fistula (ROOF).

His contrast enema is shown in Figures 4.2 through 4.4.

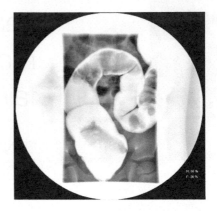

Figure 4.3 Contrast enema, frontal view, showing the rectosigmoid.

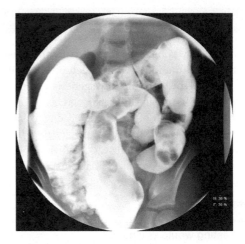

Figure 4.4 Contrast enema, frontal view, showing entire colon.

The post-evacuation film is shown in Figure 4.5.

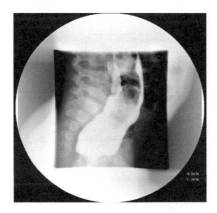

Figure 4.2 Contrast enema, lateral view.

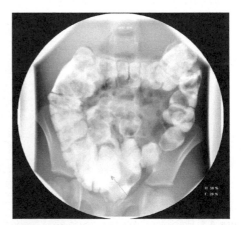

Figure 4.5 Post-evacuation film.

QUESTION 4.4

What does the contrast study show?

Answer: The contrast study shows a redundant rectosigmoid colon. The post-evacuation film shows partial emptying of colonic contrast with residual contrast remaining throughout the colon.

Upon exam in the clinic, the patient had a slight posteriorly located anoplasty. His spinal MRI revealed him to have a fatty filum without tethering. His sacral ratio is AP: 0.41, Lat: 0.69. The renal ultrasound showed normal kidneys with a mild post-void residual, and a 2 cm cystic structure adjacent to the posterior right aspect of the urinary bladder.

QUESTION 4.5

What do you think this cystic structure could be?

A. Possibly a remnant of the original fistula (ROOF)
B. A bladder stone
C. A ureterocele

Answer: The pelvic MRI confirmed the suspicion that this cyst was in fact a very small remnant of the original distal rectum attached to the posterior urethra (Answer = A). This did not require any surgical intervention.

QUESTION 4.6

What would the patient's potential for bowel continence be?

A. Good
B. Fair
C. Poor

Answer: The ARM Index is a tool utilized to help gauge an individual's level of bowel continence. It is based on a number system which categorizes individuals into good, fair, or poor potential for continence (refer to the figure "ARM Index" in the color insert).

This patient's ARM type is a rectoprostatic fistula (2 points). His spine revealed abnormal fatty thickening of filum, which adds an additional 2 points. His sacral ratio is 0.69, which will bring his final number to 6. Based on utilizing the ARM Index, this patient's potential for bowel continence is fair (Answer = B).

QUESTION 4.7

What regimen would you start?

A. Rectal enemas
B. Continue current regimen of MiraLAX, lactulose, and Fleet enemas
C. Laxatives and fiber
D. Bisacodyl

Answer: Based on his first evaluation, he was placed on rectal enemas (Answer = A). These were started because the colon shows distention and the child was having frequent stool accidents. This would indicate that he is not on the correct bowel regimen at present. The patient was not started on a laxative and fiber regimen because his colon needed time to shrink down to a manageable size. If the colon is too distended when you start a laxative and fiber regimen, the dose needed to provoke a proper bowel movement would be a higher dose. Starting with a higher dose could cause an increase in abdominal cramping, which could deter the patient from continuing the medication in the beginning.

QUESTION 4.8

Why are rectal enemas typically started first?

Answer: If the patient has good or fair potential for bowel continence, rectal enemas are a way to reset the colon to allow for the colon distention to shrink to a normal sized colon. Giving the rectal enemas for 6 to 12 months will allow this to occur. Starting with rectal enemas is a "quick fix" to help promote social continence. The patient begins to learn what it is like to be clean and not have stool accidents. This will provide the patient with motivation if laxatives and fiber are tried in the future.

BOWEL MANAGEMENT WEEK

DAY 0

Patient report:

- Regimen: 1 cap MiraLAX twice a day, 2 tablespoons lactulose daily, a Fleet enema as needed
- Family reports 1–2 accidents per day and 1 voluntary bowel movement every other day with the help of a Fleet enema (Figure 4.6)

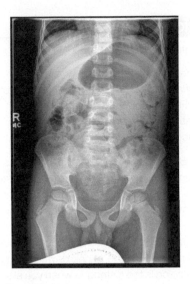

Figure 4.6 Day 0 X-ray.

The recommended regimen to start bowel management was 500 mL normal saline and 30 mL glycerin based off the contrast volume amount and to stop the MiraLAX, lactulose, and Fleet enemas.

DAY 1 OF RECTAL ENEMAS

Patient report:

- Regimen: 500 mL normal saline and 30 mL glycerin
- Voluntary bowel movement before nightly enema
- One accident 2 hours after the enema
- No complaints of pain or cramping (Figure 4.7)

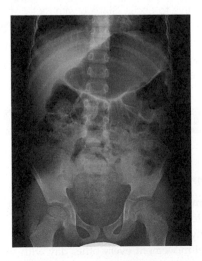

Figure 4.7 Day 1 X-ray.

22

> ### QUESTION 4.9
>
> **What does the X-ray show?**
>
> **Answer:** The X-ray shows stool distending the colon from the cecum to the rectum.

DAY 2

Patient report:

- Regimen: 500 mL normal saline, 30 mL glycerin, and 9 Castile soap
- No reported accidents (Figure 4.8)

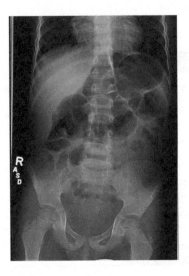

Figure 4.8 Day 2 X-ray.

> ### QUESTION 4.10
>
> **What does the X-ray show?**
>
> **Answer:** The X-ray shows an increase in gas, but a decrease in stool.

> ### QUESTION 4.11
>
> **What would you change about the regimen?**
>
> A. Continue the current regimen
> B. Stop glycerin and increase Castile soap
> C. Stop Castile soap
> D. Switch Castile soap to baby soap

Answer: The regimen was changed to 500 mL normal saline and 27 mL Castile soap. The glycerin was stopped and the Castile soap was increased (Answer = B) because glycerin can cause an increase in gas in some patients.

Answer: The normal saline was decreased to help strengthen the concentration of the Castile soap since the patient had a small overnight accident (Answer = C). The new regimen is 450 mL normal saline and 27 mL Castile soap.

DAY 3

Patient report:

- Regimen: 500 mL normal saline and 27 mL Castile soap
- Family reported one small overnight accident
- Family reported a decrease in abdominal cramping (Figure 4.9)

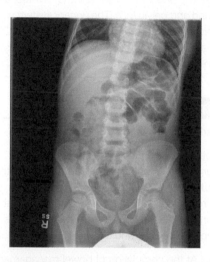

Figure 4.9 Day 3 X-ray.

DAY 4

Patient report:

- Regimen: 450 mL normal saline and 27 mL Castile soap
- Small accident reported a half hour after rectal enema
- Small overnight accident reported (Figure 4.10)

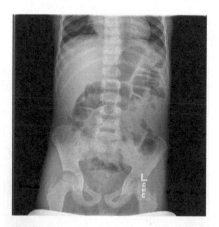

Figure 4.10 Day 4 X-ray.

QUESTION 4.12

What does the X-ray show?

Answer: Less gas is seen on this X-ray. Stool is in the ascending and transverse colon.

QUESTION 4.13

What would you change the regimen to?

- A. Continue the same regimen
- B. Change Castile soap to baby soap
- C. Decrease the normal saline
- D. Add glycerin back into the regimen

QUESTION 4.14

What does the X-ray show?

Answer: The X-ray shows stool throughout the colon in the ascending, descending, and rectum.

QUESTION 4.15

What do you want to do with the regimen?

- A. Continue the same regimen and review administration technique
- B. Decrease normal saline
- C. Change Castile soap to baby soap
- D. Decrease Castile soap and review administration technique

Answer: The administration technique was reviewed with the family and the Castile soap was decreased because the patient continued to have small accidents (Answer = D). The actual technique performed with rectal enemas is important. If one area during the administration process, that is, infusion rate of the solution, hold time of the solution, or not sitting on the toilet for the recommended 45 minutes, is performed differently than the recommendations of the health care provider, this can make the enema ineffective.

DAY 5

Patient report:

- Regimen: 450 mL normal saline and 18 Castile soap
- Small accident overnight (Figure 4.11)

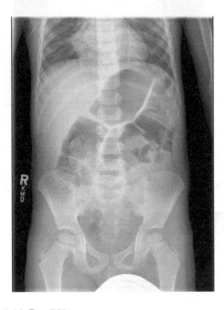

Figure 4.11 Day 5 X-ray.

QUESTION 4.16

What does the X-ray show?

Answer: The X-ray shows stool throughout the colon in the ascending, descending, and rectum. There is no change in stool volume compared to the previous X-ray.

QUESTION 4.17

What would you change the regimen to?

A. Continue the same regimen
B. Change the Castile to baby soap
C. Decrease the normal saline

Answer: The regimen was changed to 400 mL normal saline and 18 mL Castile soap. The normal saline was decreased (Answer = C) because the patient was still experiencing accidents. Decreasing the normal saline should help make the flush less diluted and the flush stronger.

An exam under anesthesia with cystoscopy was performed during bowel management week to assess the anatomy and to look for a ROOF hinted at on the ultrasound and pelvic MRI. The urinary system was found to be normal and there were no signs of a ROOF. The anus was posteriorly mislocated (outside the sphincter mechanism) by 2 cm.

QUESTION 4.18

What are the next steps?

A. Nothing, no surgical intervention is needed
B. Surgical intervention is needed to relocate the anus and create a Malone appendicostomy
C. Surgical intervention is needed to relocate the anus
D. Surgical intervention is needed for a Malone appendicostomy and Mitrofanoff only

Answer: At the completion of bowel management week, the patient was scheduled for a reoperation (redo) via a posterior sagittal anorectoplasty (PSARP) approach to move the anus to the center of the sphincters and a laparoscopic Malone appendicostomy to allow for antegrade flushes (Answer = B). During bowel management week, the patient started to resist undergoing the rectal enemas. It was decided to proceed with the Malone appendicostomy because this patient would most likely need to be on either a rectal enema regimen or an antegrade regimen to help keep him be clean of stool accidents throughout the day for longer than a 6-month period. The patient received urology clearance to proceed with the Malone only. The patient did not need a Mitrofanoff, because his urological system was normal and he was experiencing no symptoms that would indicate this intervention. Therefore, there was no need to consider that the appendix would be needed one day to be shared for a Malone and Mitrofanoff.

QUESTION 4.19

Why was a regimen started before the redo?

Answer: It is important to have a good regimen for the patient prior to the redo PSARP and Malone appendicostomy to allow the patient to begin to have social continence quickly and to allow the colon to begin to decrease in size.

A PSARP with a Malone appendicostomy was performed a few months after the completion of bowel management week. At a 1-year follow-up with the patient, the regimen was 500 mL normal salin, 30 mL glycerin, and 27 mL Castile soap. The family reported no accidents with this regimen and the patient was tolerating the antegrade flushes well. A few years later after being on antegrade flushes, the family asked to transition to laxatives. When the patient is older they can "listen" to their body as to when it is time for a bowel movement.

QUESTION 4.20

What would your next steps be?

A. The patient needs more time on antegrade flushes
B. Attend a laxative bowel management week

Answer: The patient attended a formal laxative trial during a bowel management week (Answer = B). At the beginning of the week, the patient's regimen consisted of 75 mg of ex-lax once a day with 3 g of Nutrisource fiber twice a day. At the completion of this bowel management week, the regimen consisted of 125 mg of ex-lax daily with 9 g of Nutrisource in the morning and 6 g of Nutrisource in the evening.

PRESENT DAY

During a follow-up visit, the family reported that the patient was taking 137.5 mg of senna tablets per day and 7.5 g of Nutrisource fiber twice a day. The patient was having four to six small voluntary bowel movements per day. The family reported that every one to two weeks, the patient will go 24 hours without a bowel movement and then will proceed to have several accidents for a few days. The family also reported that they will do an antegrade flush if there has been no stool output within 24 hours.

The plan for the patient is to continue their current laxative dosage and increase the fiber dosage to 9 g twice a day. The family is to do an antegrade flush once a week in the hope of "resetting" the colon to help decrease the number of accidents.

QUESTION 4.21

When do you consider switching back to antegrade flushes?

Answer: This decision is up to the family on when or if they would like to switch back to antegrade flushes, in this case possibly a more reliable way to keep the patient clean.

QUESTION 4.22

When do you discuss with the family the patient's quality of life with stool accidents?

Answer: This is a continued discussion with the family through clinic appointments, emails, and via phone calls. Psychology should be consulted based on provider discretion.

KEY LEARNING POINTS

1. If the colon shows distention on the contrast study, rectal enemas are started to help the colon shrink down to a normal size. This is done over a 6- to 12-month period.
2. Normal saline can be decreased to help strengthen the regimen by concentrating the additives.
3. Administration technique is important to review with families at the beginning of bowel management week and when they go home in order to set them up for success.

SUGGESTED READING

Reck-Burneo, C. A., Vilanova-Sanchez, A., Gasior, A. C. et al. 2018. A structured bowel management program for patients with severe functional constipation can help decrease emergency department visits, hospital admissions, and health care costs. *Journal of Pediatric Surgery*, 53, 1737–1741.

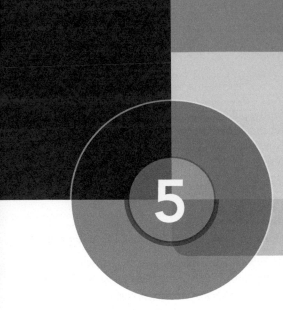

A patient with a good anatomic anorectal malformation (ARM) repair, but with poor potential for bowel control

5

CATHERINE TRIMBLE

CASE HISTORY

A 5-year-old male presents to your clinic with a history of an anorectal malformation (ARM). As a newborn, a colostomy was opened and he had a rectourethral (bladder neck) fistula for which a laparoscopic-assisted posterior sagittal anorectoplasty (PSARP) was performed. Thereafter, the colostomy was closed. The parents were told the child would be fine and no routine follow-up or any other treatments were necessary. At age 5, the child presents to you with daily soiling.

QUESTION 5.1

What do you predict is the cause of the soiling?

Answer: The most likely reason for soiling in an ARM patient would be incomplete emptying due to an ineffective bowel regimen. Essentially, for his whole life, constipation has not been worried about or managed. Also, given his malformation with a high rectum at the bladder neck, poor continence is expected. A full evaluation and workup should be completed to determine the best plan for the patient.

The mother, on her own and based on advice from a social network group, placed the patient on a daily rectal enema regimen of 350 mL of saline and 15 mL of glycerin. After being placed on these daily enemas, the child was clean and able to wear normal underwear. The patient and family are interested in transitioning from enemas to laxatives.

QUESTION 5.2

What evaluation do you suggest?

Answer: Spinal MRI, sacral X-rays, exam under anesthesia, contrast enema.

Spinal MRI reveals termination of the conus at L4, consistent with a tethered cord. Neurosurgery evaluated him for this and performed a cord detethering.

Sacral ratio AP: 0.58; lateral: 0.66.

Examination revealed an anus well centered within the sphincter complex, with no stricture or prolapse.

A contrast enema via the rectum was obtained (Figure 5.1)

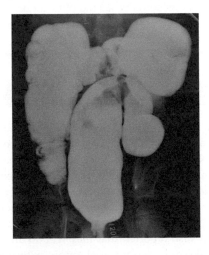

Figure 5.1 Contrast enema.

QUESTION 5.3

How do you interpret the findings on the contrast enema?

Answer: Dilated ascending, transverse, and descending colon. Significantly distended rectum and distal sigmoid colon. Sigmoid redundancy.

QUESTION 5.4

Why do you think the colon looks this way?

Answer: The dilation is due to years of constipation and inadequate colonic emptying.

QUESTION 5.5

According to the ARM continence predictor index, what is the patient's potential for bowel control (refer to the figure "ARM Index" in the color insert)?

Answer: His original malformation is a recto–bladder neck fistula (3 points), his conus terminates at L4 (tethered cord, underwent release) (2 points), and he has a sacral ratio of 0.66 (2 points). Therefore, the patient has poor potential for bowel control (7 points in total).

Despite the prediction of having a poor potential for continence, the patient and family desired to trial transitioning from rectal enemas to laxatives. The patient was started on senna, 45 mg once daily with 3 g of water soluble fiber twice a day (BID). Rectal enemas were stopped (Figure 5.2).

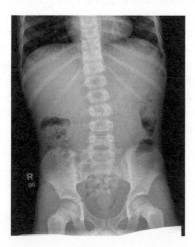

Figure 5.2 Abdominal X-ray, Bowel Management Day 2.

The patient reported seven voluntary bowel movements and one stool accident in the last 24 hours. Five of the voluntary bowel movements were within 2 hours of each other.

QUESTION 5.6

What is your assessment of the X-ray?

Answer: There is stool in the ascending and transverse colon. The descending colon and the rectum are empty.

QUESTION 5.7

Based on the X-ray and the stooling report from the patient, what regimen changes would you make?

Answer: The bowel regimen changes were:

- Continue senna, 45 mg daily
- Increase water soluble fiber to 6 g BID

The laxative dose that the patient is on is properly emptying his colon of stool. The patient reports multiple bowel movements in a 24-hour period. The increase in water soluble fiber should work to consolidate the number of stools the patient is having (Figure 5.3).

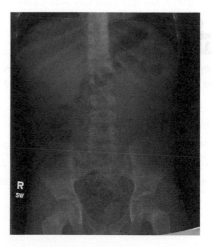

Figure 5.3 Abdominal X-ray, Bowel Management Day 3.

On day 3 of bowel management the patient reported three small, soft voluntary bowel movements with three stool accidents in the last 24 hours. The patient had not had a bowel movement yet prior to the X-ray. His current bowel regimen was senna, 45 mg daily with water soluble fiber, 6 g BID.

QUESTION 5.8

What changes would you make to this patient's bowel regimen based on the X-ray and report from the last 24 hours?

- **A.** Continue the same regimen
- **B.** Increase laxatives
- **C.** Decrease laxatives
- **D.** Increase fiber
- **E.** Decrease fiber

Answer: The senna was increased to 60 mg once daily (Answer = B) due to stool accumulation throughout the colon on the X-ray. The increase in senna will also help the patient empty more effectively with the goal being one to two formed bowel movements per day.

The patient's regimen was changed to senna, 60 mg daily with fiber, 6 g BID. The patient reported five soft, formed voluntary bowel movements with two stool accidents in the last 24 hours. The patient is having four stools in the morning; both accidents were in the afternoon. The abdominal X-ray from the day was clean.

QUESTION 5.9

What regimen changes can you make to decrease the number of stools the patient is having a day?

- **A.** Decrease laxatives
- **B.** Increase laxatives
- **C.** Add loperamide

Answer: The patient's previous regimen was 45 mg of senna, which was not enough to empty his colon, so you

do not want to decrease the laxative dose. The patient has a clean X-ray, an increased dose would cause more stooling and more accidents. Loperamide can be added to help quiet the colon (Answer = C), provide some bulk to the stool, and prevent accidents.

The patient's regimen is changed to senna, 60 mg daily, fiber 6 g BID and loperamide 1 mg in the morning. He did not have a bowel movement for 22 hours after the loperamide, and he had increased stool in the colon on the X-ray. His loperamide dose was decreased to 0.5 mg in the morning.

The regimen at the end of bowel management week was senna, 75 mg daily with fiber, 6 g BID. The loperamide was stopped because it caused too much bulk. The patient continued to struggle, having several voluntary stools a day and several accidents a day.

QUESTION 5.10

Other than loperamide, what can be done to decrease the number of stools the patient is having?

Answer: A dose of water soluble fiber can be added during the day to add bulk and consolidate the stool to decrease the number of stools a day.

A dose of fiber was added in the middle of the day. The patient's regimen was then senna, 75 mg daily with fiber 6 g in the morning and evening and 3 g in the afternoon. The patient continued to report multiple stools a day with multiple stool accidents a day. Despite several changes to both the laxative and fiber, a regimen was not found that effectively emptied the colon and produced one to two well-formed stools a day with no accidents. Essentially, we were unable to find the "sweet spot"—the combination of diet, fiber, and senna that produce one to two well-formed stools per day with control. The decision was made to return to rectal enemas.

QUESTION 5.11

What else can be done for this patient?

Answer: The option of a Malone appendicostomy can be offered to this patient to allow for an antegrade approach for enemas. An antegrade enema option will allow the patient to be independent as he gets older (Figure 5.4).

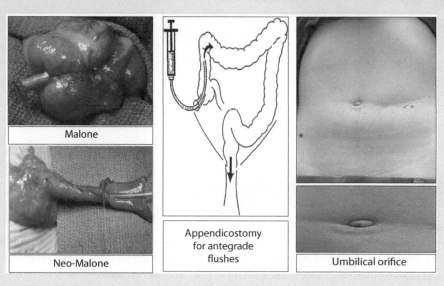

Malone

Neo-Malone

Appendicostomy for antegrade flushes

Umbilical orifice

Figure 5.4 (See color insert.) Malone appendicostomy.

KEY LEARNING POINTS

1. The patient and family's goals and wishes need to be evaluated and taken into consideration when making decisions regarding bowel regimens.
2. Patients with poor potential for bowel control can potentially be successful on a laxative regimen and should be allowed to trial laxatives if desired. If they are not successful, a mechanical regimen is needed and a Malone offers a comfortable antegrade option which allows for independence.
3. Peristeen and a sacral nerve stimulator are also considerations for this patient which could tip them over into continence. (This is the subject of a future chapter.)
4. An increased number of daily bowel movements on a laxative regimen can mean several things. It can mean that a patient is overstimulated, requiring a decrease in the laxative dose. It can also mean that the patient is understimulated and is stooling small amounts without fully emptying the colon. Additionally, it could mean that the stool needs to be bulked and consolidated, which can be achieved with water soluble fiber. An X-ray helps differentiate between the possibilities.

SUGGESTED READINGS

Lawal, T. A., Rangel, S. J., Bischoff, A., Pena, A., & Levitt, M. A. 2011. Laparoscopic-assisted malone appendicostomy in the management of fecal incontinence in children. *Journal of Laparoendoscopic and Advanced Surgical Techniques*, 5(21), 455–459.

Rangel, S. J., Lawal, T. A., Bischoff, A., Chatoorgoon, K., Louden, E., Pena, A., & Levitt, M. A. 2011. The appendix as a conduit for antegrade continence enemas in patients with anorectal malformations: Lessons learned from 163 cases treated over 18 years. *Journal of Pediatric Surgery*, 46(6), 1236–1242.

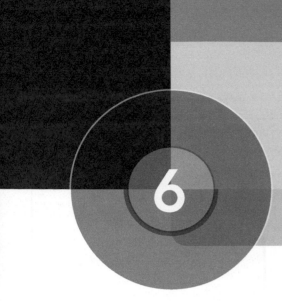

6

A patient with a history of a cloacal malformation who needs colorectal, urological, and gynecological collaboration

KRISTINA BOOTH

CASE HISTORY

A 5-year-old female with a history of cloacal malformation, was previously repaired at an outside hospital and also had a tethered cord release as an infant. She presents to your clinic for bowel management and a multidisciplinary evaluation by colorectal, urology, and gynecology.

This patient wears a diaper for both stool and urine. From the colorectal standpoint, she is taking polyethylene glycol 3350 17 g once daily. She has significant perineal skin breakdown due to frequent loose stools. From the urological perspective, the patient is incontinent of urine and denies feeling the sensation to void. She has a history of afebrile urinary tract infections every 6 months and is treated regularly by her primary care provider for these with oral antibiotics. The family is motivated for the patient to be clean of stool and dry of urine, and they report that the patient has never had a gynecological assessment.

QUESTION 6.1

What initial workup would you recommend for this patient?

Answer: Workup included:

- Examination under anesthesia, which showed a well-positioned and properly sized anus.

- Cystoscopy showed a trabeculated bladder. The urethra was 4.2 cm in length and was catheterizable with an 8F coude catheter.
- Vaginoscopy showed a vagina with evidence of a previously resected vaginal septum and two normal appearing cervices.
- Lateral sacral ratio of 0.5.
- A contrast enema via the rectum is shown in Figure 6.1.

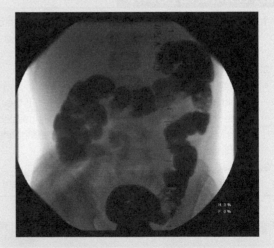

Figure 6.1 Contrast enema.

QUESTION 6.2

What would be your colorectal plan for bowel management based on this information?

A. No change to her bowel regimen
B. Start an oral laxative
C. Start an enema regimen

Answer: C. Given the patient's history of cloaca, tethered cord, and sacral ratio of 0.5, she has poor potential for bowel control. She will likely not be successfully continent for stool on an oral laxative regimen, as she has been treated with thus far. Therefore, she would benefit from a daily enema regimen, a mechanical program to empty her colon once per day.

- Urological evaluation included a renal ultrasound and voiding cystourethrogram as part of the video urodynamics.

The renal ultrasound showed right Society of Fetal Urology (SFU) grade 3 hydronephrosis with a dilated ureter and left SFU grade 2 hydronephrosis.

Video urodynamics are shown in Figures 6.2 and 6.3.

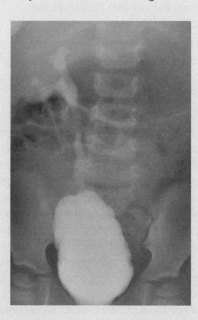

Figure 6.2 Video urodynamics imaging.

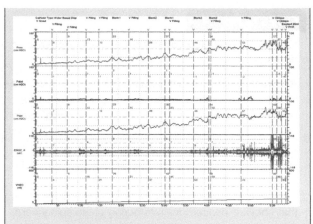

Figure 6.3 (See color insert.) Urodynamics.

QUESTION 6.3

What is your interpretation of the video urodynamics?

A. Normal urodynamics
B. Smaller than expected bladder capacity, but low detrusor pressures with normal bladder compliance. Normal appearing bladder seen on the video portion with right grade 3 vesicoureteral reflux (VUR)
C. Reduced bladder compliance, small bladder capacity and elevated detrusor pressures. Trabeculated bladder on video portion with right grade 3 VUR

Answer: C. The urodynamics showed a smaller than expected bladder capacity. The patient's estimated bladder capacity using the Koff formula [(age in years + 2) × 30 = bladder capacity in mLs] is 210 mL, her actual bladder capacity was 80 mL. There was also reduced bladder compliance with elevated detrusor pressures up to 63 cm H_2O. Elevated detrusor pressure is defined as pressures over 40 cm H_2O and may put a patient at risk for upper tract deterioration. On the video portion, the bladder appeared trabeculated and there was right grade 3 VUR. These video urodynamic findings are concerning for future upper urinary tract deterioration.

QUESTION 6.4

Who might you also consult given these urodynamic findings?

Answer: Given the urodynamic findings of reduced bladder compliance and high detrusor pressures, neurosurgery was consulted. The neurosurgical team often uses urodynamic findings to help guide their decision-making regarding a tethered cord. Specifically, neurosurgery is looking for bladder changes or bladder deterioration noted on the urodynamics.

A repeat spinal MRI was also completed on this patient that showed concern for retethering of the spinal cord. Given the MRI and urodynamic findings, the neurosurgery team recommended surgery to re-release the tethered cord.

QUESTION 6.5

What was the goal of the tethered cord re-release?

Answer: The goal of the tethered cord re-release was to prevent continued deterioration of bladder/bowel function and nerve function.

QUESTION 6.6

While awaiting the tethered cord surgery, what would you recommend for the colorectal and urological plans?

Answer:

Colorectal: The patient was started on a daily rectal enema program. She completed bowel management with a regimen of 400 mL of saline and 25 mL of glycerin. On this regimen she was having no fecal soiling, the enema time was 1.5 hours, and her abdominal X-rays showed no significant stool accumulation after her enema.

Urological: Given the urodynamics findings with reduced bladder compliance and elevated detrusor pressures, the patient was started on clean intermittent catheterization every 3–4 hours to empty the bladder and an anticholinergic medication to help improve bladder filling pressures. Our plan is to repeat a renal ultrasound and urodynamics in 3 months after the retethered cord release.

QUESTION 6.7

Why do we wait at least 3 months after a tethered cord release to repeat urodynamics testing?

Answer: There is a period of spinal shock initially after the tethered cord release, so to assess long term bladder function it is best to wait at least 3 months to reassess the bladder dynamics.

Follow up (3 months later):

Colorectal: The patient continued with rectal enemas. Her regimen is 400 mL of saline and 30 mL of glycerin. She started to have minimal soiling in between enemas each day and began to have a longer flush time of 2.5 hours. We increased the strength of her enema regimen to try to improve colonic emptying, but the patient developed abdominal cramping and did not tolerate this increased regimen.

QUESTION 6.8

What could you offer this patient?

   A. Antegrade option, such as Malone appendicostomy
   B. Antegrade option and colon resection
   C. No change to bowel regimen

Answer: B. We discussed a Malone appendicostomy and the potential for a colon resection given the lengthy enema time and the patient not tolerating a more concentrated enema regimen. One can anticipate that a sigmoid resection will improve the flush time by about 1 hour.

Urological: Repeat urological testing 3 months after starting catheterizations and while on an anticholinergic showed improving right SFU grade 2 hydronephrosis and dilated ureter and stable left SFU grade 2 hydronephrosis. Her urodynamics showed increased bladder capacity of 190 mL (expected capacity of 210 mL) and improved bladder compliance with a maximum detrusor pressure of 25 cm H_2O (previously had maximum detrusor pressure of 63 cm H_2O). It is important to note the improvement to the upper urinary tract is directly a result of improved bladder management. Aggressive and proactive treatment to ensure bladder emptying and safe bladder filling pressures can prevent upper tract changes and chronic kidney disease.

The patient was not tolerating urethral catheterizations well and catheterizations proved to be difficult. The patient was dry in between catheterizations when catheterized every 4 hours.

QUESTION 6.9

How would you proceed?

A. Appendicovesicostomy

B. Appendicovesicostomy and bladder augmentation

C. Appendicovesicostomy with bladderneck procedure to increase outlet resistance

Answer: A. The urological plan was for an appendicovesicostomy, given the patient was not tolerating urethral catheterizations well. Since the patient's repeat urodynamics showed improved bladder capacity and improved bladder dynamics, there was no need to consider a bladder augmentation. The patient was also dry in between catheterizations, thus she did not require any bladder outlet procedure.

After a collaborative discussion with the colorectal, urological, and gynecological teams, the plan we formulated was to perform a Malone appendicostomy and appendicovesicostomy using a split appendix technique and sigmoid resection. If the urology team felt a bladder augmentation was necessary, the sigmoid colon that is already being resected could be used for the bladder augmentation. The gynecology team also planned to perform an inspection of Mullerian structures at the time of this reconstructive surgery, as this is an ideal time to confirm gynecological anatomy and allow for proper planning of menstruation and future obstetrical potential.

Intraoperative: The patient underwent surgery and had a Malone appendicostomy and appendicovesicostomy using the split appendix technique (Figures 6.4 and 6.5)

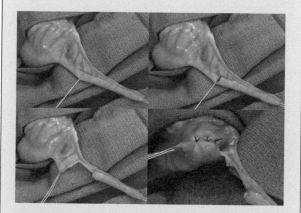

Figure 6.4 (See color insert.) Split Malone appendicostomy.

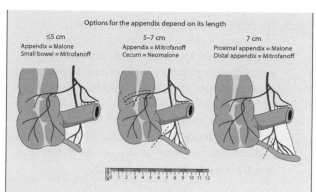

Figure 6.5 Options for the appendix.

and a sigmoid colon resection. The gynecology team also did an inspection that showed normal bilateral fallopian tubes and ovaries and two uterine horns.

Postoperative follow up and plan: The patient did well, postoperatively.

Colorectal: The patient's antegrade flush was adjusted to 400 mL of saline and 10 mL of glycerin. For the first month this was given as 200 mL of saline and 5 mL of glycerin twice a day before being combined into a single flush. Her flush time was reduced to 45 minutes and she is not having any soiling in between her flushes.

Urological: The patient is catheterized per appendicovesicostomy every 3–4 hours and doing well. She is on an anticholinergic daily and remains dry in between catheterizations. She has not had any urinary tract infections and is scheduled for routine renal ultrasounds for follow up to monitor for upper urinary tract changes.

Gynecological: The patient will have a pelvic ultrasound 6 months after thelarche. Normal menses and good obstetric potential are anticipated.

KEY LEARNING POINTS

1. It is important to do an initial thorough assessment when evaluating a patient with complex ARM. This initial assessment should include a colorectal evaluation, urological evaluation, and gynecological evaluation.

2. For patients with a history of tethered cord, it is important to have a neurosurgical assessment if there are urological symptoms. It is helpful to have both a repeat spinal MRI and urodynamics to help guide the neurosurgeon's decision-making.

3. For patients who have completed bowel management with enemas who are unable to tolerate the amount of stimulants required to empty the colon or have a longer flush time, a colon resection (of the sigmoid colon) should be considered.

4. Patients with complex ARM should be cared for by a multidisciplinary team. Often, surgeries are able to be coordinated together to eliminate additional anesthetics with this team approach.

SUGGESTED READINGS

Eradi, B., Hamrick, M., Bishoff, A., Frischer, J. S., Helmrath, M., Hall, J., Pena, A., & Levitt, M. A. 2013. The role of a colon resection in combination with a Malone appendicostomy as part of a bowel management program for the treatment of fecal incontinence. *Journal of Pediatric Surgery*, 48(11), 2296–300.

Pradhan, S., Vilanova-Sanchez, A., McCracker, K. A., Reck, C. A., Halleran, D. R., Wood, R. J., Levitt, M. A., & Hewitt, G. D. 2018 November. The Mullerian Black Box: Predicting and defining Mullerian anatomy in patients with cloacal abnormalities and the need for longitudinal assessment. *Journal of Pediatric Surgery*, 53(11), 2164–2169.

Koff, S. A. 1983 March. Estimating bladder capacity in children. *Journal of Urology*, 21(3), 248.

Vanderbrink, B. A., Levitt, M. A., Defoor, W. R., & Alam, S. 2014 April. Creation of an appendicovesicostomy Mitrofanoff from a preexisting appendicocecostomy utilizing the split appendix technique. *Journal of Pediatric Surgery*, 49(4), 656–659.

Vilanova- Sanchez, A., Halleran, D. R., Reck-Burneo, C. A. et al. 2019 March. A descriptive model for a multidisciplinary unit for colorectal and pelvic malformations. *Journal of Pediatric Surgery*, 54(3), 479–485.

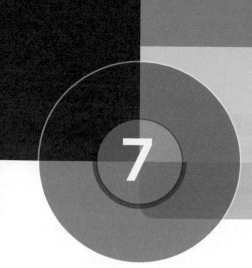

A young adult with prior surgery for an anorectal malformation (ARM) with fecal incontinence

ONNALISA NASH

CASE HISTORY

A 25-year-old female with a history of a complex cloaca comes to your clinic. She underwent cloacal reconstruction with a posterior sagittal anorectovaginourethroplasty (PSARVUP) as a baby and subsequently underwent a redo of her repair with partial vaginal replacement with rectum several years later due to an inadequate perineal body and introital stenosis. She underwent a Malone appendicostomy at age 5 to provide for antegrade access for flushes. Over time, she continued to require more concentrated and voluminous daily flushes to empty. The flush volume and additives were being increased by the nursing team regularly and the flush was taking longer than an hour and a half. Her Malone leaks stool 1 to 2 times per week. She presents to you for evaluation for help with improving her bowel management regimen. Her Malone flush currently is 200 mL saline, 30 mL glycerin, and 30 mL Castile soap, then 200 mL saline 10 minutes after administration. She also takes Colace 100 mg daily. She continues to experience stool accidents daily and prolonged emptying. Her urological history includes chronic kidney disease (CKD) stage 1–2, bladder and kidney stones, hydronephrosis, and bilateral vesicoureteral reflux. She catheterizes per urethra and is dry between cathing.

QUESTION 7.1

Which two evaluations from the following list would be pertinent to initially assess this patient?

A. Examination under anesthesia (EUA)/cysto/
vaginoscopy
B. Anorectal manometry
C. Colonic manometry

D. Contrast enema
E. Sitz marker study

Answer: A and D.

A is important to evaluate the position and anatomy of her anal opening, as well as the location and quality of her urethra and vagina.

D is important to evaluate the anatomy of her colon including location, length, and diameter.

EVALUATION

- *EUA/cysto/vaginoscopy:* Anus well-positioned and without stricture; the cystoscopy and vaginoscopy were unremarkable
- Magnetic resonance imaging (MRI) of the spine revealed sacral dysplasia and no tethered cord
- Contrast enema is shown in Figure 7.1

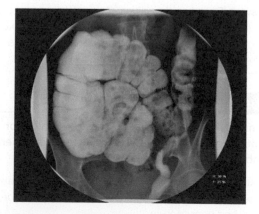

Figure 7.1 Final image of contrast enema.

- Sacral ratio: AP 0.3 and lateral 0.39 (Figure 7.2 and refer to the figure "ARM Index" in the color insert)

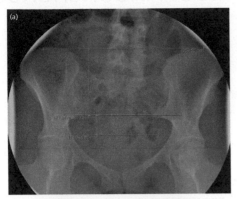

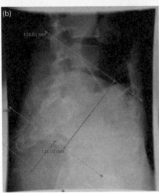

Figure 7.2 (a) AP X-ray image of sacrum and (b) lateral image of sacrum.

QUESTION 7.2

Are these sacral ratios poor, fair, or good?

Answer: Based on the values of sacral ratio poor (<0.4), fair (0.4–0.7), and good (>0.7), this sacral ratio would be considered poor, and represents significant caudal regression.

QUESTION 7.3

Considering the ARM index as a predictor of continence, what would you predict is this patient's probability for continence?

Answer: The patient has a poor to intermediate probability for continence, due to a high type of malformation, normal spine, and poor sacrum.

QUESTION 7.4

After assessing this contrast study how would you describe the colon?

Answer: The contrast study reveals a narrowed segment of the distal aspect of the descending colon.

Note: It is important to assess the anatomy in order to troubleshoot any problematic flush by simulating the flush using the Malone and performing an antegrade study.

QUESTION 7.5

What do you think this narrowing represents?

Answer: This is likely due to ischemia at the area of the previous colostomy closure and/or area of colonic vaginal interposition.

QUESTION 7.6

Knowing this segment is narrowed, what would your next step be?

    A. Increase strength of flush to help improve emptying
    B. Surgery to resect the narrowed segment
    C. Add loperamide to slow transit of distal colon
    D. Colonic manometry to assess motility of distal colon

Answer: B (surgical intervention).

- We decided to perform an exploratory laparotomy, colonic resection of the narrow-left colon, and Malone revision due to leaking stool from the Malone. Of note, the rectal pull-through was widely patent. The area of narrowing began at the distal left colon and reached to the peritoneal reflection. This was the area we resected. Her surgery went well. The left colon was quite narrow but a healthy transverse colon was successfully anastomosed to the neo rectum, which was normal caliber.

Postoperatively, the patient was on twice daily flushes for 1 month then was transitioned to Malone flushes with saline 300 mL and glycerin 20 mL. Her flushes were initially improved after surgery, but over time the length of flush increased. She contacted our center with concerns that the flush was taking over 2 hours. An abdominal X-ray was obtained (Figure 7.3).

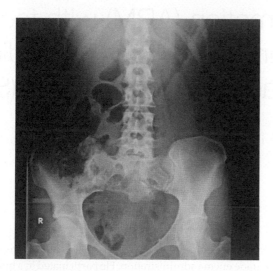

Figure 7.3 Abdominal X-ray.

The X-ray now shows a clean colon. The flushes are working and the patient is clean.

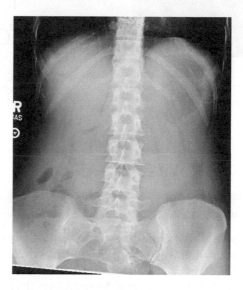

Figure 7.4 Abdominal X-ray after flush adjustment.

QUESTION 7.7

In a patient with the X-ray shown in Figure 7.3 and extended flush time, what change should be made to the flush?

A. Increase saline
B. Increase glycerin
C. Decrease glycerin
D. Decrease saline

Answer: A and B.

Change Malone flushes to saline 350 mL and glycerin 30 mL to increase volume and strength due to stool in descending colon. The current flush was not emptying the colon well.

Her follow up X-ray is shown in Figure 7.4. The patient is now doing well with no soiling and the flushes are taking around 1 hour.

KEY LEARNING POINTS

1. The initial workup is invaluable, especially the EUA and contrast imaging. Simulating the flush with an antegrade contrast study is vital.
2. A long flush time can mean a few things, including: (1) the flush is not a large enough volume to make it through the colon; (2) the flush is too strong and is causing continued contractions of the colon; (3) the flush is not strong enough and is not emptying the colon; (4) there is an anatomic blockage impeding the flush; and/or (5) there is reflux of the flush into the terminal ileum (discussed in a subsequent case). Abdominal X-rays help to clarify which case you are dealing with.

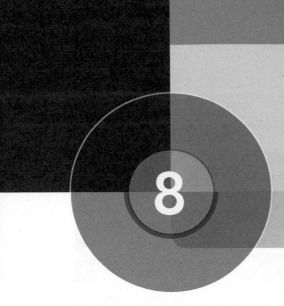

8

A patient with an anorectal malformation (ARM) with fecal incontinence who is a candidate for a sacral nerve stimulator (SNS)

CATHERINE TRIMBLE

CASE HISTORY

A 12-year-old male presents to your clinic with a history of an anorectal malformation (ARM). The original malformation is unknown. He was initially managed with a colostomy and underwent a posterior sagittal anorectoplasty (PSARP) and colostomy closure in his first year of life. He subsequently underwent two reoperations for anterior mislocation of his anus and a stricture, as well as a Malone appendicostomy for antegrade enema administration. He participated in a bowel management program to determine the ideal flush regimen. His current antegrade flush regimen is saline 500 mL, glycerin 30 mL, and Castile soap 5.5 mL. He is clean on this regimen with only occasional stool accidents (one to two per month). The patient is interested in transitioning from antegrade flushes to laxatives.

QUESTION 8.1

Which of the following diagnostic tests would you want to obtain to predict continence potential?

A. Abdominal X-ray
B. MRI spine
C. MRI pelvis
D. Contrast enema

E. Sacral X-ray
F. Colonic motility

Answer: B and E.

The potential to be continent is based on three factors: the type of anorectal malformation that a patient has, the quality

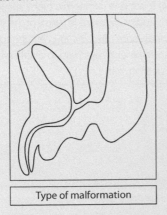
Type of malformation

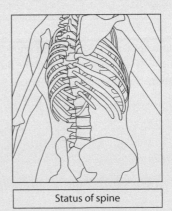
Quality of sacrum

Status of spine

Figure 8.1 Predictors of continence in ARM.

of the patient's spine, and the quality of their sacrum (ARM continence index) (Figure 8.1).

The type of malformation should be known from the initial imaging and operative findings at the time of the initial ARM repair. The sacral X-ray will provide information regarding the quality of the sacrum and objectively assess the degree of caudal regression. An MRI of the spine provides information on the quality of the patient's spine and assesses for tethered cord.

EVALUATION

- Original malformation is unknown
- Sacral ratio AP: 0.64, lateral: 0.84
- Normal MRI of the spine, no evidence of tethered cord

Examination of the perineum revealed an anus located within the sphincter complex, no prolapse or stricture, and good sphincter contractions were noted.

QUESTION 8.2

Using the ARM continence predictor index, what is the patient's potential for bowel control (refer to the figure "ARM Index" in the color insert)?

Answer: The MRI was normal (1 point). The lateral sacral ratio was 0.84 (1 point). The original malformation is unknown, but the patient appeared to have had a good repair with good sphincter muscles. Total points: 3–5. Therefore, the patient has a good potential for bowel control. He should be successful on laxatives and no longer need antegrade flushes.

The plan was to have him participate in a bowel management week to transition from antegrade enemas to laxatives.

QUESTION 8.3

What diagnostic test would you want to obtain prior to beginning bowel management?

- **A.** Colonic motility
- **B.** Contrast enema
- **C.** Abdominal X-ray

Answer: B. The contrast enema allows the provider to fully assess the colon, noting the colonic anatomy and degree of colonic distention. It provides valuable information that helps guide the choice for the starting bowel regimen (Figure 8.2).

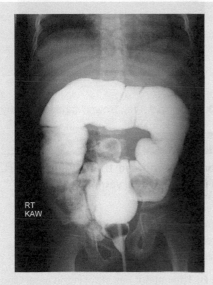

Figure 8.2 Contrast enema, Bowel Management Day 1.

QUESTION 8.4

What is your assessment of the contrast enema? What would your starting bowel regimen be?

Answer: The patient has a somewhat dilated colon without redundancy. He should be able to empty well, but will most likely need stimulant laxatives.

Based on the contrast study, it was determined that the patient should be started on a moderate dose of stimulant laxatives. Water-soluble fiber was also started to add bulk and form to the stool. The patient was started on senna 45 mg and 3 g of water-soluble fiber twice a day (BID) (Figure 8.3).

On bowel management day 4, the patient's regimen is senna 37.5 mg (2.5 squares) with water-soluble fiber 4 g BID. The patient reports several bouts of diarrhea and soiling overnight.

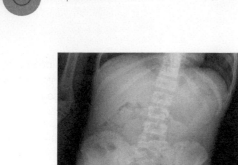

Figure 8.3 Abdominal X-ray, Bowel Management Day 4.

QUESTION 8.5

Based on the X-ray and the patient's report, what regimen changes would you make?

A. Increase laxatives
B. Decrease laxatives
C. Increase fiber
D. Decrease fiber

Answer: B. The patient has stool in the ascending colon and has a report of several stools with soiling accidents but mostly controlled bowel movements. This could indicate that the laxative dose is too high and the patient is being overstimulated. The decision was made to decrease the laxative dose.

The regimen was changed to senna 30 mg once daily with 4 g of water-soluble fiber BID (Figure 8.4).

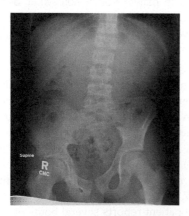

Figure 8.4 Abdominal X-ray, Bowel Management Day 7.

Regimen is 22.5 mg (1.5 squares) with 5 g of water-soluble fiber BID. Patient reports eight stools in 24 hours with one accident overnight.

QUESTION 8.6

How would you manage this patient moving forward?

A. Continue current dose of senna and fiber
B. Continue to adjust senna and fiber
C. Resume previous regimen of Malone flushes
D. Resume previous regimen of Malone flushes and consider a sacral nerve stimulator (SNS)

Answer: D. The laxative trial was not successful. For now, going back to flushes makes the most sense to get the patient clean again. The SNS can help patients who have done well on an enema regimen, but have been only partially successful transitioning to laxatives. The SNS can help by improving anal canal sensation and/or sphincter control.

The patient continued to have multiple stools a day with soiling despite several regimen changes. The patient and the family believed that the patient's quality of life was better while on antegrade flushes. The decision was made to resume the patient's previous bowel regimen. Essentially, with more laxatives, the colon empties but the patient does not have adequate bowel control. When the laxative dose is lowered, then the patient does not stool, and the "sweet spot" whereby the right amount of laxative and fiber provide the stool consistency needed for continence cannot be achieved. Therefore, the patient needs a mechanical regimen. It is in just such a case that SNS could have a valuable role.

QUESTION 8.7

What information and testing would you need before proceeding with the SNS?

Answer: Colonic manometry (CMAN) would be needed to assess for colonic dysmotility and in this case showed normal motility throughout most of the colon with lower motor activity in the distal third of the colon.

Anorectal manometry (AMAN) is vital to assess baseline rectal sensation and the patient's ability to squeeze, and in this case showed an intact rectoanal inhibitory reflex

(RAIR), normal anal sphincter pressure, and good squeeze pressure. Therefore, no outlet procedures are needed such as botulinum toxin or biofeedback.

Sacral X-rays, to understand the degree of caudal regression and for SNS procedure planning, were already obtained.

An MRI of the pelvis and spine were already obtained to assess for any spinal anomalies or indications for a redo PSARP, such as a remnant of the original fistula.

The decision was made to trial an SNS and a temporary lead was placed. An AMAN was repeated 4 days later, which showed improved rectal sensation. The patient reported that he was able to sense stool in his rectum and that he was able to have controlled bowel movements between his flushes.

The patient did well with the temporary SNS and a permanent SNS was inserted 1 month later. The patient then returned for bowel management to transition from rectal enemas to laxatives.

A repeat contrast enema, now 1 year after the previous one, was obtained (Figure 8.5).

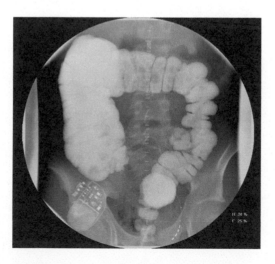

Figure 8.5 Contrast enema, Bowel Management Day 1.

Contrast enema via the Malone prior to starting bowel management showed improved peristalsis in the left colon as indicated by haustral markings. He was started on senna 45 mg and water-soluble fiber 2 g three times a day (TID).

This X-ray was obtained after starting senna and holding flushes (Figure 8.6).

Day 7 of bowel management week: The regimen was senna 75 mg once daily with 1 g of water-soluble fiber TID. The patient reported one to two formed bowel movements a day with no soiling accidents.

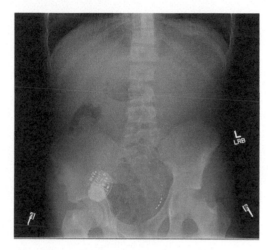

Figure 8.6 Abdominal X-ray, Bowel Management Day 7.

KEY LEARNING POINTS

1. Despite having a good potential for bowel control, the patient was initially unable to transition from antegrade enemas to laxatives.
2. Patients with ARM may benefit from an SNS if they desire to be continent on laxatives and have potential for continence. SNS can "tip them over the edge" into continence. It has also been shown to improve the antegrade flush, and is known to improve urinary/bladder function as well.
3. It is important to understand the patient's and family's goals when discussing bowel management and future options.

SUGGESTED READING

Sulkowski, J. P., Nacion, K. M., Deans, K. J., Minneci, P. C., Levitt, M. A., Mousa, H. M., Alpert, S. A. & Teich, S. 2015. Sacral nerve stimulation: A promising therapy for fecal and urinary incontinence and constipation in children. *Journal of Pediatric Surgery*, 50(10), 1644–1647.

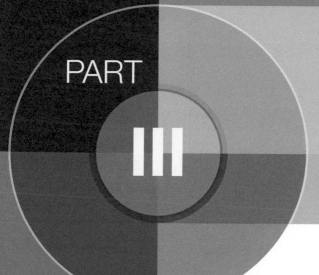

PART III

HIRSCHSPRUNG DISEASE

INTRODUCTION

Stacie Leeper

Hirschsprung disease (HD) is a congenital malformation in which the nerves (ganglion cells) in the colon do not form properly. The incidence of HD is approximately 1 in 5,000 live births. These nerves are responsible for peristalsis; therefore, patients with HD develop functional intestinal obstruction starting at the level at which the nerves failed to migrate. The bowel downstream from the ganglion cells is unable to relax, therefore this distal segment remains contracted leading to a functional obstruction. The level of aganglionosis can occur anywhere in the colon and, in rare cases, even involve the entire colon and small bowel (total intestinal HD). The most common type typically affects the left colon or sigmoid colon.

HD usually presents in the newborn period when the infant does not pass meconium in the first 48 hours of life. The infant with HD may also have abdominal distention, explosive, foul-smelling stools, bilious emesis, feeding intolerance, or failure to thrive. This presentation of enterocolitis results from the stasis of stool leading to bacterial overgrowth. The bacterial overgrowth can then lead to translocation (the process by which bacteria crosses into the bloodstream through cracks in the intestinal mucosa) which can make the patient very ill. Older children diagnosed with HD often present with chronic constipation.

If HD is suspected in the newborn period, rectal irrigations should be initiated to decompress the colon. During a rectal irrigation, a soft tube is passed into the rectum and the colon is gently "washed" with small volumes of saline. The goal of rectal irrigation is to remove stool and gas from the bowel and prevent stasis of stool in the colon. Once the colon is adequately decompressed, contrast enema should be performed. The classic finding of HD on contrast enema is a transition zone between the normal and aganglionic bowel (see Figure III.1).

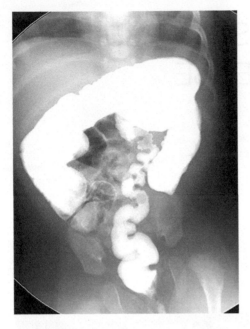

Figure III.1 Decompressed bowel in the rectosigmoid, dilated bowel up to the left colon, the transition zone is suspected to be in the proximal sigmoid.

Another helpful diagnostic tool for children over 1 year of age is the use of anorectal manometry to evaluate for recto-anal inhibitory reflex (RAIR). The RAIR is reflexive relaxation of the internal anal sphincter in response to rectal dilation and is found to be absent in children with HD. Anorectal manometry is useful in the evaluation of an older child who suffers from chronic constipation. In this case, if the RAIR is present, the diagnosis of HD can be ruled out, therefore eliminating the need for rectal biopsy. If RAIR is absent, HD must be confirmed with rectal biopsy. If the biopsy is normal the patient may have internal sphincter achalasia, which will be discussed in a subsequent chapter.

The gold standard for definitive diagnosis is a rectal biopsy that demonstrates the absence of ganglion cells in the submucosa as well as the presence of hypertrophic nerves. In the newborn period, a suction rectal biopsy can be done, however full-thickness biopsy is necessary in children over 1 year of age. Once the diagnosis has been made, the definitive treatment is surgical. The goal of surgical management is to remove the aganglionic segment of the bowel and bring the normally innervated segment down to the anus. The anal sphincters and anal canal must be preserved in order for the child to achieve future continence. The three most commonly performed

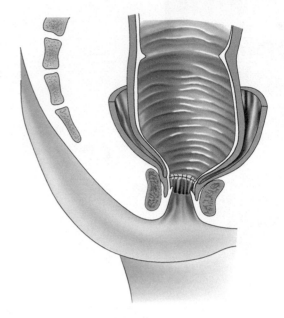

Figure III.2 Soave technique.

operations for HD are the Soave, Swenson and Duhamel procedures (see Figures III.2–III.4). The Soave pull-through removes mucosa and submucosa of the rectum, and the ganglionated bowel is pulled down and placed within a cuff of the aganglionic muscle. The Swenson

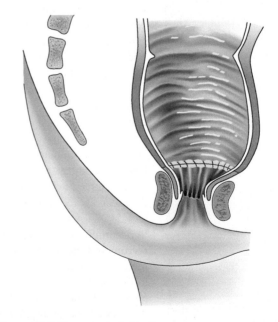

Figure III.3 Swenson technique.

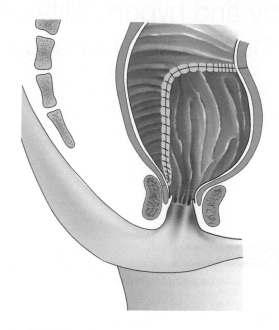

Figure III.4 Duhamel technique.

pull-through removes the entire aganglionic segment of the bowel, with an end to end anastomosis above the anal sphincter. In the Duhamel procedure, the normal colon is brought down through the plane between the rectum and the sacrum. The two walls are joined to create a new lumen that is aganglionic anteriorly and normally innervated on the posterior side. In all cases, the anal canal should be carefully preserved. Therefore, if surgery is done well, the abnormal smooth muscle (internal) sphincter remains intact, which can have clinical implications later.

The complications that can occur after pull-through surgery can typically be placed in one of the two following categories: (1) obstructive or (2) soiling. Obstructive symptoms include abdominal distention, vomiting or episodes of enterocolitis, similar to a newly diagnosed case of HD. Children with enterocolitis in the postoperative period present with abdominal distention, fever, vomiting, feeding intolerance and foul-smelling explosive stool. Chronic enterocolitis and obstructive symptoms can lead to failure to thrive. Treatment for enterocolitis includes rectal irrigations, hydration and metronidazole (Flagyl). Obstructive symptoms can be caused by the mechanical obstruction from a stricture, a twist in the pull-through,

an obstructing Soave cuff, a transition zone pull-through or a large Duhamel pouch. If none of these are present, the non-relaxing sphincter can be the problem.

The second category of complication following a pull-through procedure is soiling. Soiling can be due to damage to the sphincter or dentate line during the original operation. A surgeon must be meticulous in protecting these structures so that a child is not left with injured continence mechanisms. Soiling can also occur with intact sphincters and dentate line when the colon either moves too quickly (hypermotility) or too slowly (hypomotility). This can be treated medically by creating a good bowel movement pattern with the goal of one to two soft, formed stools per day, either by speeding up or slowing down the stooling.

Children with HD naturally have "tight" anal sphincters that do not relax normally. While they are still young, many may need botulinum toxin injection into the anal canal until they are old enough to learn how to overcome that sphincter on their own which will allow them to empty their colon successfully. Botulinum toxin can be repeated as frequently as every 3 months as necessary.

SUGGESTED READINGS

Frykman, P. K. & Short, S. S. 2012. Hirschsprung-associated enterocolitis: Prevention and therapy. *Semin Pediatr Surg.* 21(4),328–35.

Koivusalo, A. I., Pakarinen, M. P., & Rintala, R. J. 2009. Botox injection treatment for anal outlet obstruction in patients with internal anal sphincter achalasia and Hirschsprung's disease. *Pediatric Surgery International* 25(10),873–876.

Langer, J. C., Rollins, M. D., Levitt, M. et al. 2017. Guidelines for the management of postoperative obstructive symptoms in children with Hirschsprung disease. *Pediatric Surgery International* 33(5),523–526.

Levitt, M. A., Dickie, B., & Pena, A. 2010. Evaluation and treatment of the patient with Hirschsprung disease who is not doing well after a pull-through procedure. *Semin Pediatric Surgery* 19, 146–53.

Levitt, M. A., Dickie, B., & Pena, A. 2012 Nov. The Hirschsprung patient who is soiling after what was considered a "successful" pull-through. *Semin Pediatric Surgery* 21(4), 344–53.

9

A patient with good surgical anatomy and hypomotility after a Hirschsprung pull-through

LEAH MOORE

CASE HISTORY

A 3-year-old female with Hirschsprung disease and significant developmental delay presents with persistent constipation and overflow soiling.

Originally, the patient was diagnosed at 2 years of age with Hirschsprung disease with a transition zone in the rectosigmoid and underwent a primary Swenson pull-through. The X-ray done on her first follow-up visit 1 month after her pull-through is shown in Figure 9.1.

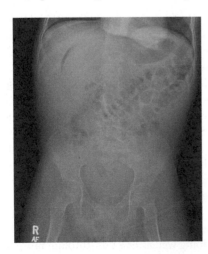

Figure 9.1 Abdominal X-ray at the one month visit.

QUESTION 9.1

What does this X-ray show?

Answer: No colonic distention post–pull-through, no retention of stool.

QUESTION 9.2

What would be your recommended plan?

Answer: The patient was advised to irrigate for any distention. No stooling medications were recommended.

The patient returned at 2 months and her mother reported that the patient was feeling well, eating well, and had resumed all normal activities. She was having three loose bowel movements a day and there had been no need for irrigations. An X-ray was performed (shown in Figure 9.2).

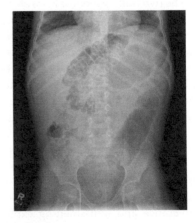

Figure 9.2 Abdomal X-ray.

QUESTION 9.3

What does this X-ray show?

Answer: Moderate retained stool throughout the colon and a mildly dilated pull-through.

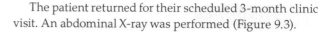

QUESTION 9.4

What would be your recommended treatment?

Answer: The X-ray shows retention of stool and gas. We were concerned about three things: (1) an anastomotic stricture; (2) obstruction from her non-relaxing sphincters; and (3) a slow-moving colon in need of laxatives. Because of this, the patient underwent an exam under anesthesia to confirm that there was no stricture (and none was found). The dentate line and sphincter complex were both intact. Botulinum toxin was administered into the internal sphincter to paralyze the non-relaxing internal anal sphincters, with the idea that as the botulinum toxin effect wears off over several months the child would "learn" to stool on their own, by pushing to overcome the non-relaxing sphincters.

QUESTION 9.5

What would be your plan now?

Answer: To treat a slow-moving colon, once we confirmed there was no anatomic problem with the pull-through, we started the patient on 30 mg of senna daily to help to stimulate the bowel to move. In order to help consolidate and bulk the stool, we added 3 grams of water-soluble fiber twice per day and waited for the botulinum toxin to start to work.

WATER-SOLUBLE FIBER

Refer to Table 9.1.

The patient returned for their scheduled 3-month clinic visit. An abdominal X-ray was performed (Figure 9.3).

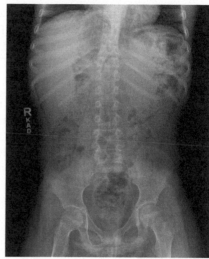

Figure 9.3 Abdominal X-ray.

QUESTION 9.6

Why did we start senna?

Answer: The patient's X-ray showed a moderate amount of stool burden along with mild dilatation of the pull-through. We concluded that the patient was not emptying effectively and needed the help of a stimulant laxative.

Table 9.1 Water solube fiber options.

Type	Dosage and use	Where to find it
Pectin (Sure-Jell)	1 tablespoon = 2 g of fiber	Found in the grocery store in the jelly/canning section or online at www. pacificpectin.com. Get the sugar-free version.
Citrucel (methylcellulose)	*Powder* 1 tablespoon = 2 g of fiber *Capsule* 2 capsules = 1 g of fiber	Found in the pharmacy section of the store or online at www.citrucel.com. You can use the generic or the brand name. Get the sugar-free version.
Metamucil (psyllium husk)	*Powder* 1 teaspoon = 2 g of fiber *Capsule* 5 capsules = 2 g of fiber *Wafer* 1 packet (2 wafers) = 3 g of fiber	Found in the pharmacy section of the store or online at www.metamucil.com. Get the sugar-free version.
Nutrisource (guar gum)	1 tablespoon (scoop) = 3 g of fiber *(Can be sprinkled on food or mixed in drinks.)*	Found in the pharmacy section of the store, online, or through homecare companies.

QUESTION 9.7

What does this X-ray show?

Answer: There is formed stool throughout in the ascending, transverse, and sigmoid segments. There is mild distention of a stool-filled rectum.

Stooling report:

- Senna 30 mg once daily; the mother had not been giving the recommended water-soluble fiber, instead choosing to give "high fiber foods"
- Three to four loose, runny bowel movements daily
- No irrigations have been done due to the patient not having any distension
- No fever, foul-smelling stool, straining to stool, cramping, nausea, or vomiting

QUESTION 9.8

Based on this report, what would you suggest?

Answer: We increased the senna to 45 mg once daily and encouraged the mother to give the recommended 6 g of supplemental water-soluble fiber twice per day. The family was to send a stooling report in 1 week. The plan was for them to follow up in clinic in 2 months with an X-ray prior.

Most recently, the mother reports difficulty with getting the child to take the fiber regimen. The patient is having 3–4 loose bowel movements per day. The mother reports no concerns for any obstructive symptoms. We encouraged her to continue to incorporate the fiber regimen into the diet as much as possible.

QUESTION 9.9

What is the rationale behind adding water-soluble fiber to the stimulant laxative?

Answer: Stimulant laxatives can cause watery stools if not given with a water-soluble fiber. We use a water-soluble fiber to help absorb the water in the stool and create bulk to the stool.

KEY LEARNING POINTS

1. Laxatives can only be effective in this case because the patient has an anatomically correct pull-through and has the capacity to achieve voluntary bowel movements.
2. Starting laxatives are sometimes needed to help effectively empty the colon and help prevent colonic dilation resulting from stool retention.
3. Water-soluble fiber is also needed in conjunction with the laxative therapy to help bulk and create good consistency of stool. The key to success is to obtain a good bowel movement pattern; that is, one to two well-formed stools per day.
4. Compliance with the fiber regimen can be a challenge particularly in children with a diagnosis of developmental delay.
5. Botulinum toxin is used to paralyze (force relaxation) of the inherently non-relaxing sphincters of patients with Hirschsprung disease. This is only given to patients with an intact dentate line.

10

A patient with good surgical anatomy and hypermotility after a redo pull-through for Hirschsprung disease

LEAH MOORE

CASE HISTORY

A 3-year-old male with a history of Hirschsprung disease underwent a colostomy creation as a newborn and then a pull-through of his colostomy. His parents have had to do daily rectal irrigations for distention and the lack of spontaneous bowel movements. The patient also had three enterocolitis episodes requiring hospital admission post–pull-through.

QUESTION 10.1

What would you do for an evaluation of these symptoms?

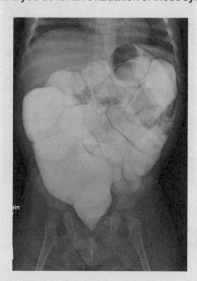

Figure 10.1 Contrast enema.

Answer: Exam under anesthesia, rectal biopsy, and contrast enema were planned as part of his initial evaluation. The exam under anesthesia was to assess anatomy and the previous surgery. Rectal biopsies were needed to assess for the presence of ganglion cells and to check whether this was a transition zone pull-through. A contrast enema was performed to evaluate the pull-through (Figure 10.1).

QUESTION 10.2

What do you see?

Answer: The image demonstrates that the colon pull-through comes down the right pelvis. There is very little colon (essentially, he only has his right colon) and mild dilation of the pull-through. The bowel opacified by the contrast on the left side is all small bowel.

An exam under anesthesia revealed no twist or stricture. The rectal biopsy showed an absence of ganglion cells and there were hypertrophic nerves.

QUESTION 10.3

What is your interpretation of those results and what would be your plan be, given these findings?

Answer: These findings are consistent with a transition zone pull-through. Based on these results and the obstructive symptoms, we performed a redo transanal pull-through for retained transition zone. The ganglionic bowel was found 6 cm higher in the colon. Thereafter, we planned to have the patient return in 1 month for an examination under anesthesia to assess the anastomosis.

One month after the redo, the patient's mother reported 9 to 10 stools per day in the weeks following surgery, resulting in extensive perineal skin breakdown. There was no further distention or any obstructive symptoms.

QUESTION 10.4

Do you think the redo was successful?

Answer: Yes—his obstructive symptoms have been eliminated. Now he is suffering from loose stools, which can be medically managed. And, this should be anticipated given how little colon he has.

QUESTION 10.5

What would your plan of action be?

Answer: Obtain an abdominal image to assess stool burden. The abdominal X-ray is shown in Figure 10.2.

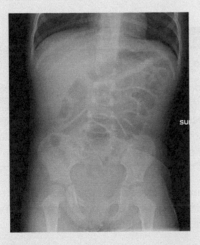

Figure 10.2 Abdominal X-ray.

QUESTION 10.6

What do you see?

Answer: The X-ray image showed no stool, and no gaseous distension.

QUESTION 10.7

Based on patient's report and X-ray assessment, would this patient be hypermotile or hypomotile?

  A. Hypermotile

  B. Hypomotile

Answer: Hypermotile. We concluded this based on the mother's stooling reports of 9 to 10 liquid bowel movements (BMs) per day and no stool seen on X-ray image. He also has a severe perianal rash.

QUESTION 10.8

Given the conclusion of hypermotility, what would your plan be?

Answer: The plan was to begin adding water-soluble fiber to consolidate and bulk his stool, and decrease his frequency to a goal of two to three BMs per day. This also will improve the skin breakdown.

The patient presented for a planned 1-month exam under anesthesia.

X-ray prior to exam under anesthesia is shown in Figure 10.3.

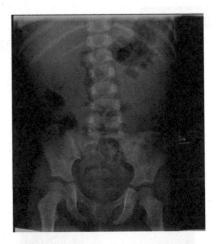

Figure 10.3 Abdominal X-ray.

QUESTION 10.9

What do you see?

Answer: There is mild to moderate formed stool in the rectum.

The patient underwent a planned 1-month exam under anesthesia. The anal canal and sphincter complex were intact. The anastomosis had healed well with no stricture.

No Botulism toxin was given. It was clear we were now successfully bulking the stool.

QUESTION 10.10

What would your plan be now?

Answer: The plan was to increase the amount of fiber based on the stooling reports of liquid stools. The goal is to achieve more stool bulk. Education on a constipating diet was provided and recommended (Tables 10.1 and 10.2).

Table 10.1 Constipating diet phase 1

Food group	Food recommendations	Foods to avoid or limit
	Phase 1	
Milk	Plain rice milk	All others
Vegetables	None	If vegetables are eaten, make sure they are cooked and not raw
Fruits	Applesauce, apples (without skin), bananas	Avoid raw fruits
Starch, grains	White flour, refined flour	All others
	Bread, crackers, pasta and noodles, white rice, white potatoes (without skin),dry cereals	
Meat, seafood, legumes	Baked/broiled/grilled meats, poultry or fish, lean deli meats, eggs	Avoid beans
Fats, oils	Nonstick spray, nonfat butter spray	Limit butter, margarine, and oils No fried foods
Sweets	Sugar-free gelatin, popsicles, jelly, or syrup Rice-milk ice cream	All others
Beverages	Water, Gatorade, sugar-free Crystal Light, sugar-free Kool-Aid, Pedialyte	Avoid carbonated beverages, soda, juices, high-sugar drinks

Table 10.2 Constipating diet phase 2

Food group	Food recommendations	Foods to avoid
	Phase 2	
Milk	All milk products allowed, but limit to 500 mL (16 oz) total per day	Any milk or cheese product (such as ice cream) with nuts or seeds
Vegetables	Vegetable juice without pulp Vegetables that are well cooked Green beans, spinach, pumpkin, eggplant, potatoes without skin, asparagus, beets, carrots	Raw vegetables Vegetables with seeds
Fruits	Applesauce, apples (without skin), banana, melon, canned fruit, fruit juice (without pulp)	Fruit juice with pulp, canned pineapple, prunes, dried fruit, jam, marmalade
Starch, grains	Bread, crackers, cereals made from refined flours Pasta or noodles made from white flours White rice, pretzels, white potatoes (without skin), dry cereal	Whole-grain or seeded breads Whole-grain pasta Brown rice, oatmeal bran cereal, whole-grain cereal

(continued)

Table 10.2 (Continued) Constipating diet phase 2

	Phase 2	
Food group	**Food recommendations**	**Foods to avoid**
Meat, seafood, legumes	Meat, poultry, eggs, seafood Baked, broiled, or grilled are preferred cooking methods	Beans Fried or greasy meats, salami, cold cuts, hot dogs, meat substitutes
Fats, oils	All oils, margarine, butter, mayonnaise, salad dressings	Chunky peanut butter, nuts, seeds, coconut
Sweets	Jelly, "Rice Dream" frozen desserts, sugar, marshmallows, angel food cake	Anything containing nuts, coconut, whole-grains, dried fruits or jams
Beverages	Water, Gatorade, sugar-free Crystal Light, sugar-free Kool-Aid, Pedialyte	Juice, regular soda, regular Kool-Aid or powdered drinks
Miscellaneous	Salt, sugar, ground or flaked herbs and spices, vinegar, ketchup, mustard, soy sauce	Popcorn, pickles, horseradish, relish, jams, preserves

We continued to increase the water-soluble fiber to the maximum dosage tolerable (4 g twice per day). At that point, the patient had achieved a good "peanut butter" consistency; however, the frequency of the stools varied between four and six stools per day.

QUESTION 10.11

What would you try to incorporate next to help with the desired goal of two to three BMs per day?

Answer: We started the patient on loperamide to help with the hypermotility and the patient's stooling patterns improved to three to four BMs per day which was acceptable to the family (Table 10.3).

Table 10.3 Loperamide dosing

Tablets = 2 mg
Max dose 0.8 mg/kg/d

2. Family compliance to reporting and implementing changes was the key to success for achieving this patient's desired bowel management goals.
3. The medications should be given at the same time every day. This is very important to a child with hypermotility to achieve a consistent stooling pattern.
4. Fiber dosings should always be split up and given throughout the day, not in a single dose.
5. Enemas can also be used to help control a fast-moving colon, help to limit soiling and improve a perianal rash.

SUGGESTED READING

Levitt, M. A., Dickie, B., & Pena, A. 2010. Evaluation and treatment of the patient with Hirschsprung disease who is not doing well after a pull-through procedure. *Seminars in Pediatric Surgery*, 19(2), 146–153.

KEY LEARNING POINTS

1. Hypermotility is common post redo pull-through. It should be treated first with a constipating diet, then water-soluble fiber, then loperamide. This process should be done over 1–2 months gradually, so as not to induce constipation.

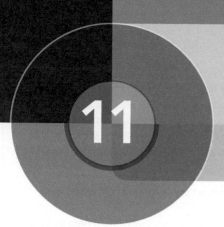

A child with Hirschsprung disease (HD) and hypomotility

11

LINDSAY REILLY

CASE HISTORY

A 4-year-old child presents with chronic constipation. In the early days of life, the child started a 4-year cycle of passing one or fewer stools per week, painful stooling, and passing a large fecal stool ball only after receiving a pediatric glycerin suppository, followed by "sandy and tarry diarrhea." She had daily abdominal distension with vomiting and decreased oral intake with each one of these "flare ups," which occurred approximately twice per month for 4 years. During that time, it was noted by the patient's pediatrician that the child had a "tight" digital rectal exam and she was referred to a gastroenterologist (GI). The child was started on polyethylene glycol 3350 (17 grams twice daily) to treat the constipation. The patient had several trips to the emergency department for abdominal pain and distension, and was always discharged with the diagnosis of "functional constipation/severe anorectal incoordination." On occasion, the child would be able to stool after a digital rectal exam in the emergency room.

QUESTION 11.1

What is the differential diagnosis?

Answer:
- Functional constipation
- Internal sphincter achalasia
- Hirschsprung disease (HD)
- Anorectal malformation (ARM)

QUESTION 11.2

What are the key facts to help narrow your differential diagnoses?

Answer:
- Tight sphincter, with pre anatomic anal stenosis
- Stooling with suppository/stooling after digital rectal exam

These two clinical findings further narrow the differential diagnoses to internal anal sphincter achalasia and Hirschsprung disease. This is due to the high internal anal sphincter pressure that is found in both disorders. The use of a suppository or the digital rectal exam functions to overcome the tight internal anal sphincter and stool is able to pass through at that time.

Before we met her she was admitted to the hospital due to a severe episode of bilious emesis. Her evaluation included an abdominal X-ray. The X-ray revealed a large amount of stool throughout the colon and gas in a nondilated small bowel.

The child underwent polyethylene glycol 3350 cleanout given via nasogastric tube, and rectal irrigations to augment stool removal. It was noted by the staff that there was a large amount of gas released when a large bore soft catheter was passed into the anus for the irrigation.

QUESTION 11.3

Why would there be so much gas released from passing a catheter into the anus?

Answer: Due to the absent rectoanal inhibitory reflex (RAIR) in HD and in internal sphincter achalasia, the internal anal sphincter squeezes tightly, trapping gas and stool in the colon. When the catheter was placed rectally, it bypassed the internal sphincter allowing the gas to escape. Due to this presentation, she was evaluated for the possibility of HD.

A biopsy was completed, but the results were still pending. A biopsy is a key piece of information in the case of refractory constipation. It determines the next course of treatment. Aganglionic bowel is incapable of receiving the impulses necessary to move stool through the colon. This process is complicated by an obstructive outlet (the internal sphincter). The result is stasis of stool and gas. Removal of the diseased bowel gives the patient the best possible anatomy and therefore, the greatest potential for normal stooling.

The patient was discharged from the hospital after the cleanout and workup, with a diagnosis of constipation, while awaiting the biopsy results.

QUESTION 11.4

What type of bowel management would you start and why?

Answer: Bowel management at this point for this patient should consist of irrigations. They should be utilized until HD is ruled out via biopsy results. This is a safety measure. An irrigation will bypass the sphincters and allow stool and gas to exit through the catheter. The addition of polyethylene glycol will thin the stool and allow it to be more easily irrigated out through the catheter. The use of large volume enemas should be avoided, as the liquid will just be retained in the colon. This will exacerbate the patient's obstructive symptoms.

QUESTION 11.5

What other imaging would be helpful and why?

Answer: A contrast enema can help map the transition zone. If the colon is significantly dilated, this is not ideal for a primary pull-through surgery, as the anastomosis

would need to be tapered. This is particularly prevalent in a patient such as this who presents at an older age. In this scenario, the patient could complete 3 months of rectal irrigations and allow the colon to shrink prior to the pull-through for a safer nontapered anastomosis (Figures 11.1 and 11.2).

- Identify the most important part of this contrast enema.
  - Inverse rectosigmoid ratio. Take note that it is not as obvious in this patient owing to the low level of the Hirschsprung disease.
- What is the presumed level of transition zone and how do you know this?
  - Presumed rectosigmoid transition zone. Presumed because the area of Hirschsprung is distal to the dilated portion. This is because the stool cannot progress through the area of aganglionated bowel and it backs up, thus dilating the colon proximal to it.

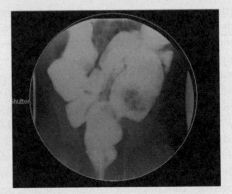

Figure 11.1 Contrast enema.

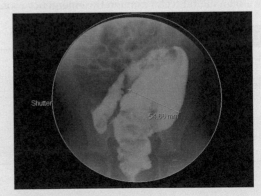

Figure 11.2 Contrast enema, post evacuation film.

The biopsy results came back 1 week later and identified prominent neural hypertrophy in the colon and rectum with no ganglion cells identified.

QUESTION 11.6

What is the diagnosis of this child's constipation?

A. Functional constipation
B. Hirschsprung disease
C. Henoch-Schonlein disease
D. ARM

Answer: Hirschsprung disease is diagnosed by this biopsy result showing aganglionic bowel (Answer B). Hypertrophic nerves in the presence of aganglionosis confirm the diagnosis.

QUESTION 11.7

What is the treatment that will provide this patient the greatest opportunity for successful continence?

A. Pull-through surgery to remove aganglionated bowel while preserving the integrity of the dentate line
B. Botulinum toxin to relax the internal sphincter
C. Long-term bowel management to regulate daily stool/soiling patterns
D. All of the above

Answer: A. A pull-through surgery to remove the diseased bowel is the most definitive treatment for this patient. Preservation of the dentate line and sphincters allows for successful continence in the future. Botulinum toxin to the internal anal sphincter is often an important adjunct in the management of HD in the postoperative period.

This patient completed daily rectal irrigations for 3 months. The contrast enema was repeated and showed a decrease in the dilation of the proximal colon. The primary pull-through surgery was completed. She had a proximal sigmoid colon transition zone. She returned 1 month later for an exam under anesthesia.

QUESTION 11.8

What is important to evaluate during the exam under anesthesia 1 month post–pull-though surgery?

Answer: It is important to evaluate for stricture, as this is the most common time to start developing one and the

easiest time to treat it. You can also give botulinum toxin if the patient is having trouble getting the stool to come out. Additionally, a dose of senna can help the hypomotility many patients with HD have.

For the last 4 months, the patient has been having daily soft bowel movements without any difficulty. Now the mother reports that she is having pain with stooling, straining to stool, and having decreased amount of stool. She is on the same daily dose of senna. Her X-ray is shown in Figure 11.3.

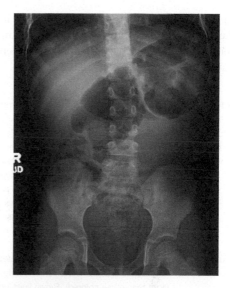

Figure 11.3 Abdominal X-ray.

QUESTION 11.9

Correlate Figure 11.3 with the clinical symptoms and provide a course of treatment.

Answer: The signs and symptoms reported are indicative of outlet obstruction and most likely caused by the tight internal sphincter associated with HD not at all surprising in this age patient. Additionally, Figure 11.3 shows stool in the descending colon and neo-rectum. The sphincter will not relax and this does not allow stool to exit. There is gas retained in the stomach and a slight amount in the ascending colon. This patient needs repeat botulinum toxin to her internal sphincter. It has been 4 months since her last injection. The botulinum toxin injection lasts on average 3 months.

QUESTION 11.10

Are there alternative treatments if she cannot get to the center to receive her injections right away?

Answer: Yes, good quality irrigations are always an option, as they bypass the internal sphincter and allow for the escape of gas and stool. It is vitally important to have the family trained in doing these, because the stasis of stool in the colon of a patient with HD can put them at high risk for Hirschsprung associated enterocolitis.

The patient returned for anal botulinum toxin injection. With the right combination of botulinum toxin injections, daily senna, and fiber, she was able to consistently and comfortably empty her colon (Table 11.1).

Table 11.1 Clinical pearls of Hirschsprung's colonic irrigations

Pearl	Rationale
Choose the right catheter.	Use the largest possible flexible catheter (a foley cather is ideal) (#24 French for older than 1 year old and #20 French for younger than 1 year old). The larger diameter allows for stool to pass through the tubing. The flexibility allows for safe deep insertion and comfortable access to stool pockets in the colon. This causes less chance of retained stool.
Irrigate until clear.	There is no set total volume for a complete irrigation. Irrigate until the fluid is nearly clear (light tea/yellow colored). Brown fluid indicates retained stool.
Irrigate using small fluid volumes.	Use small amounts (20 mL) of saline to insert repeatedly and semi-quickly to allow breakup of stool. Allow each 20 mL to drain out of catheter while moving the catheter up and down and pressing on the abdomen. Large instilled fluid volumes do not provide the pressure needed to stir up the gas and break down the stool so that it can pass through the catheter. This can leave stagnant fluid retained in the colon.
Monitor output.	Volume in = Volume out – 20 mL/kg. Retention of more than 20 mL/kg for a patient is an indication to stop the irrigation.
Change position.	The colon is a tube with twists and pockets. Twisting the catheter, changing body position and depth of the catheter insertion help to release all retained stool and pockets of gas. Abdominal massage is also helpful.

(Continued)

Table 11.1 (Continued) Clinical pearls of Hirschsprung's colonic irrigations

Pearl	Rationale
Correlate clinically.	The irrigation should release stool and gas. Evidence of successful irrigation should be decreased abdominal distension with output of gas and stool. Continued distension indicates the need for further irrigation.
Soften stool.	For frequently needed irrigations, an osmotic laxative such as polyethylene glycol 3350 can soften the stool and allow it to be more easily irrigated. Hard stool can clog the catheter.

KEY LEARNING POINTS

1. There is no substitute for a clear and well-developed history. Take the time to listen to a family and understand their course. The details in the data will often lead you to your answer. For example: Painful diarrhea, stooling with rectal exam, "tight" digital rectal exam, and large amounts of gas released when a urinary catheter is passed into the anus all point to possible Hirschsprung disease. Analysis of these key points might have led to a much earlier diagnosis.
2. Irrigations are used in HD to bypass the tight internal sphincter allowing stool and gas to escape. This helps prevent the stasis of stool and decrease the risk of enterocolitis.
3. Botulinum toxin is used to relax the internal sphincter. As it wears off, the internal sphincter will retighten and produce obstructive symptoms (painful stool passage, decreased stool, feeling urge to stool but unable, abdominal distension, gasiness).

SUGGESTED READINGS

Patrus, B., Nasr, A., Langer, J. C., & Gerstle, J. T. 2011. Intrasphincteric botulinum toxin decreases the rate of hospitalization for postoperative obstructive symptoms in children with Hirschsprung disease. *Journal of Pediatric Surgery*, 46(1), 184–187.

Tabbers, M. M., DiLorenzo, C., Berger, M. Y., Faure, C., Langendam, M. W., Nurko, S., & Benninga, M. A. 2014. Evaluation and treatment of functional constipation in infants and children: evidence-based recommendations from ESPGHAN and NASPGHAN. *Journal of Pediatric Gastroenterology and Nutrition*, 58(2), 258–274.

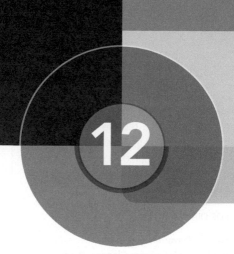

12

A patient with total colonic Hirschsprung disease and soiling

STACIE LEEPER

CASE HISTORY

A 16-month-old male presents to your clinic for an evaluation. He has a history of total colonic Hirschsprung disease (TCHD). His surgical history includes an ileostomy creation and colonic biopsies on the second day of life that confirmed the diagnosis of TCHD. He has no other significant medical, surgical, or family history. He takes one tablespoon of pectin two times per day to thicken the ileostomy stool. His parents report that they empty his ileostomy bag three times per day, his output is a pudding consistency, and they have been recording his output. You have calculated his stool output to be 15 mL/kg/d. His parents are inquiring about the timing for his definitive pull-through procedure.

It was determined that the child was a good candidate for his definitive pull-through based on the fact that he had thick output and was growing well. He went to the operating room for his ileoanal pull-through (of the ileostomy) and colectomy, via a transanal Swenson-like technique, with an abdominal incision at the ileostomy site.

QUESTION 12.1

What factors need to be taken into consideration when determining the timing of the definitive pull-through procedure in a patient with TCHD?

Answer: A patient is determined to be ready for definitive pull-through when their ileostomy output is less than 30 mL/kg/d and is thick in consistency. Thickened stool will give a child a greater chance of achieving continence, as loose stool is more difficult to control. In order to help thicken the ileostomy output, one may consider starting pectin or a water-soluble fiber. Children with an ileostomy are also at risk for failure to thrive. This is very dependent on where in the small bowel the ganglionated bowel began. It is important that a child is growing well, as adequate nutritional status is imperative for postoperative healing. In addition to monitoring a child's growth curve, it is important to check urine sodium as sodium loss is significant in a stoma and sodium facilitates glucose transport and improves nutritional absorption.

QUESTION 12.2

Knowing that the perineal skin will be exposed to small bowel contents for the first time, what treatment should be considered prior to the patient leaving the operating room?

Answer: Because the patient is at high-risk for skin breakdown, it is important be proactive with regards to skin care and apply a skin barrier such as Cavilon Advanced (3M) or Marathon (Medline).

QUESTION 12.3

After the pull-through, when thinking about bowel management, it is important to understand the motility of the colon. What type of motility do you anticipate this patient will exhibit?

A. Hypomotility
B. Normal motility
C. Hypermotility

Answer: Because this patient has no colon, they will need aggressive treatment for hypermotility.

After surgery, the patient stools well and is tolerating a regular diet after 6 days. He is ready for discharge.

QUESTION 12.4

Based on his anticipated hypermotility, what type of education should the parents receive prior to discharge with regard to the child's diet?

Answer: The parents should have the child follow a constipating diet (Figure 12.1). Diet is the first step in managing hypermotility. A constipating diet can provide bulk as well as help reduce the frequency of stooling. In particular, he should avoid high sugar food and drinks.

Food Group	Example of Constipating Foods
Milk	All milk products allowed, but limit to 500 grams (16 oz) per day
Vegetables	Vegetable juice without pulp, well-cooked vegetables, green beans, spinach, pumpkin, eggplant, potatoes without skin, asparagus, beets, carrots
Fruits	Applesauce, apples (without skin), banana, melon
Starch, grains	Bread, crackers, cereals made from refined flours, pasta or noodles made from white flour, white rice, pretzels, white potatoes (without skin), dry cereal
Meat, seafood, legumes	Baked/broiled/grilled meats, poultry or fish, lean deli meats, eggs
Fats. oils	Very limited amounts of all oils, margarine, butter, mayonaise
Sweets	Sugar-free gelatin, popsicles, jelly or syrup, rice-milk ice cream
Beverages	Water, sugar-free Gatorade, sugar free Crystal Light, sugar-free Kool-Aid, pedialyte

Figure 12.1 Constipating diet.

QUESTION 12.5

Besides diet instructions, what other education is critical prior to discharge of this patient?

A. Skin breakdown prevention/treatment

B. Laxative administration

C. Rectal enema teaching

Answer A: Because this patient is at high risk for skin breakdown, the parents should receive teaching about skin breakdown prevention and treatment seen in Figure 12.2. They should also be educated to perform frequent diaper changes.

PREVENTION OF DIAPER RASH

- Clean the skin with warm water
- Apply Remedy No-Rinse Foam Cleanser (Medline)
- Pat dry with soft, dry cloth wipe (do not use baby wipes as they can be irritating to the skin)
- After cleaning the skin, apply a protective barrier such as Cavilon No-Sting Barrier Film (3M)
- Finally, apply Proshield Plus Skin Protectant (Smith & Nephew, Inc.) on the skin

TREATMENT OF MILD DIAPER RASH

- Clean the skin with warm water
- Apply Remedy No-Rinse Foam Cleanser (Medline)
- Pat dry with soft, dry cloth wipe (do not use baby wipes as they can be irritating to the skin)
- After cleaning the skin, apply a protective barrier such as Cavilon No-Sting Barrier Film (3M)
- Apply Critic-Aid Skin Paste (Coloplast) to the skin with each diaper change

TREATMENT OF MODERATE TO SEVERE DIAPER RASH (if the skin is bleeding, wet or weepy- follow these steps)

- Clean the skin with warm water
- Apply Remedy No-Rinse Foam Cleanser (Medline)
- Pat dry with soft, dry cloth wipe (do not use baby wipes as they can be irritating to the skin)
- Apply a dusting of Stomahesive Protective Powder (ConvaTec) to clean skin
- Dab the skin with a Cavilon No- Sting Barrier Film (3M) to set the powder and create a dry surface
- Apply a layer of Ilex Skin Protectant Paste (Ilex Health Products) Allow the Ilex to dry for about 1 minute
- Cover the Ilex with a layer of Vaseline or petroleum jelly
- Wipe off any stool and petroleum jelly during each diaper change, leaving the layer of Ilex in place
- Remove the Ilex once daily by soaking in a tub of warm water

Figure 12.2 Skin care instructions.

The parents call at approximately 2 weeks postoperatively reporting that their son is having four to five loose stools per day and that he is having perineal skin excoriation. They are feeding him a constipating diet and are avoiding high sugar foods. The perineum is shown in Figure 12.3.

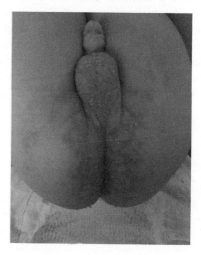

Figure 12.3 (**See color insert.**) Perineum.

QUESTION 12.6

What is your next step?

Answer: The patient is already on a constipating/low sugar diet, so the next step in hypermotility management is to start some pectin or water-soluble fiber. Pectin is a naturally occurring carbohydrate that is found in fruits and is often used as a thickening agent. Water soluble fiber binds water and helps to bulk the stool. Bulking the stool will help decrease the frequency of stool, which should in turn allow the skin to heal, because perineal irritation is related to time of stool contact on the skin.

The patient returns for his 1-month postoperative check. He is following a constipating diet and taking 2 g of water-soluble fiber twice daily. He is now having approximately eight to ten loose stools per day. He is growing well and not having any episodes of abdominal distention or fever. On physical examination, you notice his perineal area to be erythematous with skin breakdown (Figure 12.4).

His parents are following the skin care instructions that were provided to them at the time of hospital discharge (see Figure 12.2).

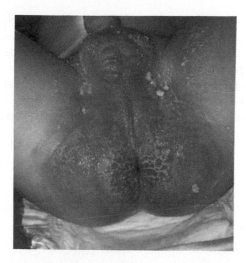

Figure 12.4 (**See color insert.**) Perineum.

QUESTION 12.7

How would you proceed with this patient given that he is having frequent loose stools despite adhering to a constipating diet and taking daily water-soluble fiber?

Answer: Because the patient is having greater than five liquid stools per day, the next step is to start loperamide (Imodium). Loperamide decreases the tone of the smooth muscle of the intestinal wall, which slows transit time allowing for greater water absorption. It is recommended that the pill form of loperamide be used as the liquid form contains glycerin as an inactive ingredient, which can stimulate the bowel and can cause more frequent stooling (Figure 12.5).

Loperamide (Imodium) dosing guide:
Tablets = 2 mg
Start at 0.25 mg/kg divided BID to TID.
Minimum dose 1 mg BID.
Max dose 0.8 mg/kg/day or 16 mg.

Figure 12.5 Loperamide dosing.

In this case, reapplication of a skin protectant (such as Cavilon Advanced, 3M or Marathon, Medline) would be beneficial. It is also important to assess the skin for a yeast rash and treat as necessary with antifungals such as nystatin powder or oral fluconazole.

Two months later, the patient returns for a follow-up clinic visit. His current regimen is a constipating diet, twice daily water-soluble fiber and loperamide three times per day (he is taking the maximum daily dose for his weight). He continues to struggle with frequent stooling (six to eight stools per day) throughout the day, but his perineal rash has dramatically improved. The perineum is shown in Figure 12.6.

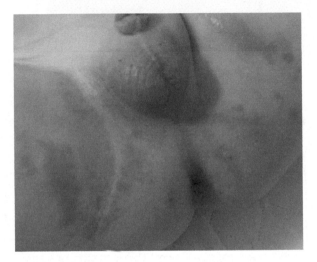

Figure 12.6 (**See color insert.**) Perineum.

QUESTION 12.8

What is the next step?

A. Stop loperamide (Imodium)

B. Start hyoscyamine (Levsin)

C. Start cholestyramine

Answer: The next step in the management of hypermotility is to add hyoscyamine (Levsin). Hyoscyamine is an anticholinergic that is used to slow the motility of the colon.

QUESTION 12.9

If you have continued difficulty managing this patient's hypermotility, what is your next step?

A. Give up

B. Consult with a gastroenterologist who is knowledgeable about short bowel syndrome

C. Suggest reopening of the ileostomy

Answer: B. Consider collaboration and consultation with GI physician who specializes in short bowel syndrome. Such providers deal with hypermotility often and can be an enormous help with these patients with Hirschsprung disease. Cholestyramine, Lomotil (Diphenoxylate + Atropine), and a clonidine patch are other treatment options that could be considered. Cholestyramine is a bile acid sequestrant and is commonly used to treat diarrhea resulting from bile acid malabsorption. Lomotil is an antidiarrheal medication that works by slowing the movement of the colon, therefore decreasing the number and frequency of bowel movements (Figure 12.7).

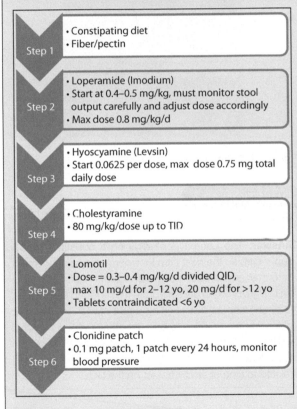

Step 1
- Constipating diet
- Fiber/pectin

Step 2
- Loperamide (Imodium)
- Start at 0.4–0.5 mg/kg, must monitor stool output carefully and adjust dose accordingly
- Max dose 0.8 mg/kg/d

Step 3
- Hyoscyamine (Levsin)
- Start 0.0625 per dose, max dose 0.75 mg total daily dose

Step 4
- Cholestyramine
- 80 mg/kg/dose up to TID

Step 5
- Lomotil
- Dose = 0.3–0.4 mg/kg/d divided QID, max 10 mg/d for 2–12 yo, 20 mg/d for >12 yo
- Tablets contraindicated <6 yo

Step 6
- Clonidine patch
- 0.1 mg patch, 1 patch every 24 hours, monitor blood pressure

Figure 12.7 Step-wise algorithm for management of hypermotility.

KEY LEARNING POINTS

1. Total colonic Hirschsprung disease can be challenging to manage in the postoperative period due to hypermotility that leads to frequent stooling and perineal breakdown.

2. Previous practice had been to delay the timing of the definite pull-through until the age of toilet training to decrease the incidence of perineal skin problems; however, if a child is able to produce stool that is applesauce consistency and is less than 30 mL/kg/d, it is now recommended to perform the pull-through between ages 6 and 18 months in order to avoid a prolonged ostomy. It is imperative that a proper bowel regimen be used in order to prevent multiple stools and skin excoriation.

3. Hypermotility is treated in a step-wise approach starting with constipating diet and water-soluble fiber.

SUGGESTED READING

O'Neil, M., Teitelbaum, D. H., & Harris, M. B. 2014. Total body sodium depletion and poor weight gain in children and young adults with an ileostomy: A case series. *Nutr Clin Pract* 29:397–401.

13

A teenager with prior surgery for Hirschsprung disease who has constipation

STACIE LEEPER

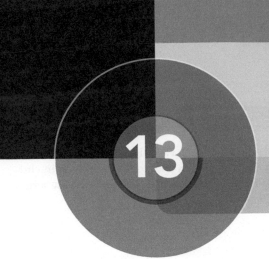

CASE HISTORY

An 18-year-old male presents to your clinic for an evaluation. He has a history of Hirschsprung disease (HD) and underwent a colostomy creation in the newborn period. He underwent a Soave pull-through of the colostomy at age 6 months. He never had any episodes of enterocolitis. Over the past few years, he has been having daily fecal soiling. He reports that he stools one to three times per day, but has smearing accidents multiple times per day. He is not currently taking any medication or supplements, but has taken senna, Colace (docusate sodium), and Dulcolax (bisacodyl) in the past with varying degrees of success.

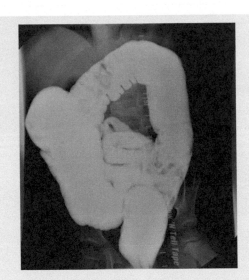

Figure 13.1 Contrast enema.

QUESTION 13.1

What is the first the first step that you will need to take to evaluate this patient?

A. Upper GI
B. Contrast enema
C. Anorectal manometry

Answer: B. A contrast enema should be obtained to evaluate the stool burden and size of the colon. Because this patient has had previous surgery for his HD, it is also important to evaluate for a twisted pull-through, colonic stricture, or problematic Duhamel pouch, although these are very unlikely given that he has not had obstructive symptoms (Figure 13.1).

QUESTION 13.2

How do you interpret the findings on the contrast enema?

Answer: The contrast enema shows a colon with the rectosigmoid absent. No stricture or twist of the pull-through is seen. The mild dilation throughout is potentially consistent with a slow-moving colon (hypomotile) and is suggestive of chronic constipation, but there are haustrations noted—which is evidence of peristalsis—therefore a colon that should respond to laxatives.

A post-evacuation film is shown in Figure 13.2.

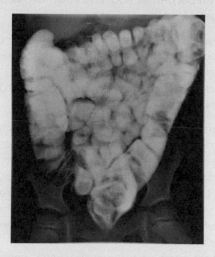

Figure 13.2 Contrast enema post-evacuation image.

QUESTION 13.3

What significant finding is revealed in the post-evacuation image?

Answer: There is retained contrast on post-evacuation evaluation further supporting the conclusion that this is a hypomotile colon.

QUESTION 13.4

Based on the findings on the contrast study, what is the next step in evaluating this patient?

A. Exam under anesthesia with rectal biopsy
B. Start patient on 17 g of MiraLAX one time per day
C. Anorectal manometry
D. All of the above
E. A and C

Answer: E. In order to fully evaluate this patient, an exam under anesthesia is imperative to evaluate the status of the anal canal (dentate line) and anal sphincters. Because this patient is soiling, anorectal manometry (AMAN) will also be helpful to further evaluate anal sphincter function.

The findings of the examination under anesthesia (EUA) are as follows: Hegar Size 18, intact dentate line (see Figure 13.3) and sphincters, no palpable cuff, twist, or stricture. Rectal biopsy results were normal (ganglion cells present with normal-size nerves).

The findings of the AMAN revealed an absent rectoanal inhibitory reflex (RAIR), normal squeeze pressure, and normal resting pressure. The exam and AMAN show that this patient underwent a technically excellent pull-through. There are no anatomic or pathologic causes of obstruction and the dentate line and sphincters were meticulously preserved.

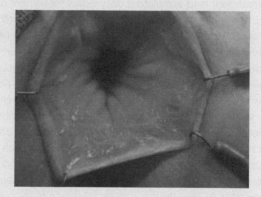

Figure 13.3 Intact dentate line observed during EUA.

QUESTION 13.5

What is your next step?

A. Botulinum toxin to the anal canal
B. Biofeedback
C. Start a stimulant laxative

Answer: C. Botulinum toxin is not indicated in this case as the patient does not exhibit high resting pressures. Biofeedback is not indicated as the patient has normal AMAN results. The patient should be started on a stimulant laxative, such as senna, to provoke the slow colon to move, and to achieve a bowel movement pattern of one to two soft, formed stools per day. For this patient, we chose to start 75 mg senna based on the size of his colon. In addition, a water-soluble fiber should be started to help bulk the stool.

QUESTION 13.6

Based on your evaluation of this X-ray as well as the patient report, what would be your next step in the management of this patient?

A. Keep his senna dose the same and stop his fiber
B. Give an over-the-counter rectal enema to "reset" the colon and then increase his senna to 100 mg per day; keep his fiber dose the same
C. Decrease his senna to 50 mg per day and keep his fiber dose the same

Answer: B. When using an oral stimulant laxative, the goal of treatment is to stimulate a daily bowel movement and empty the colon. The patient will then not have another bowel movement or soiling for 24 hours until the next treatment and will thereby be clean and able to wear normal underwear. If the patient does not stool within 24 hours, they are instructed to administer an over-the-counter rectal enema to evacuate rectal stool burden. After the enema, the laxative dose is increased. In contrast, if the patient stools multiple times and the abdominal radiograph does not have significant stool burden, the laxative dose can be decreased. In this case, the X-ray reveals a large amount of stool in the rectum. Because of this, he is instructed to administer an over-the-counter rectal enema to evacuate rectal stool burden. This will "reset" the colon. After the enema, the laxative dose is increased to 100 mg per day.

The patient returns for follow-up in 3 months. He reports little improvement in his stooling pattern since starting the senna and fiber. He is taking 75 mg senna and 4 g of water-soluble fiber every evening. He is usually having one stool per day, but sometimes goes over 24 hours without stooling. He is still having daily soiling. His X-ray is shown in Figure 13.4.

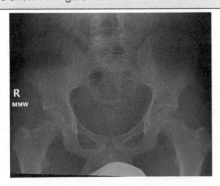

Figure 13.4 Abdominal X-ray.

QUESTION 13.7

Based on your evaluation of this X-ray as well as the patient report, what would be your next step in the management of this patient?

A. Wean him off the senna
B. Decrease his fiber dose and keep giving fiber one time per day
C. Increase his fiber dose and change its dosing to two times per day

Answer: C. His X-ray shows some stool in the rectum, but a clean left and transverse colon, so his senna dose does not need to be adjusted. Because he is still having some loose stool, it would be beneficial to increase his daily dose of fiber to help bulk his stool more. Fiber is more effective if given throughout the day, so it may help to have him take half of his dose with breakfast and the other half in the evening.

The patient returns to the clinic in 6 months and reports that he is doing well—he has achieved a stooling pattern of one to two soft, formed stools per day and is no longer having any smearing or soiling.

The patient returns for follow-up and is doing well. He is stooling one to two times per day with no accidents. He is taking 100 mg senna and 4 grams of water-soluble fiber per day. His stools are mostly soft but occasionally loose. His X-ray is shown in Figure 13.5.

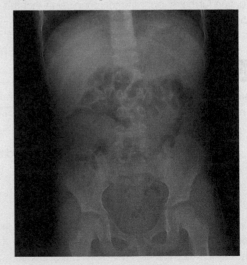

Figure 13.5 Abdominal X-ray.

KEY LEARNING POINTS

1. The problematic patient post–pull-through should be worked up in a systematic fashion to exclude all potential problems that may be causing the patient to not empty well.

2. When using an oral stimulant laxative, the goal of treatment is to stimulate a daily bowel movement and empty the colon so the patient will not have another bowel movement or soiling for 24 hours.

3. If the patient does not stool within 24 hours, they should administer an over-the-counter rectal enema to evacuate rectal stool burden and reset the colon. After the enema, the laxative dose is increased.

4. If the patient stools multiple times and the abdominal radiograph does not have significant stool burden, the laxative dose can be decreased.

SUGGESTED READING

Levitt, M. A., Dickie, B. & Pena, A. 2012. The Hirschsprung's patient who is soiling after what was considered a "successful" pull-through. *Seminars in Pediatric Surgery,* 21(4), 344–353.

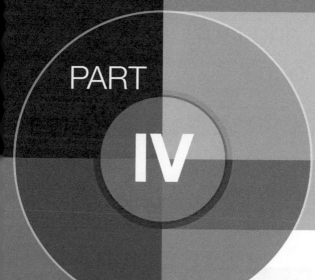

PART IV

SPINAL ANOMALIES

INTRODUCTION

Cheryl Baxter

Spinal anomalies present unique challenges for patients with regard to bladder and bowel management, with dysfunction seen commonly in patients with spina bifida (SB), sacral agenesis (SA), spinal cord injury (SCI), and diseases of the nervous system such as muscular dystrophy (MD). The bladder and rectum share an embryologic origin, have closely related autonomic and somatic innervation, and their voluntary control depends on the intact function of complex neural networks. Neurogenic bowel dysfunction (NBD) is often manifested by both fecal incontinence and constipation. The pathophysiology of NBD varies with the site and severity of the neurologic lesion.

In this section, we will discuss four case studies with varied pathophysiology related to spinal anomalies. The goal of bowel management in such patients is to accomplish complete evacuation of the rectum on a regular basis (usually mechanically with an enema program), thus reducing the risk of fecal impaction, urgency, and incontinence. Good bowel management often leads to an improvement in urinary continence.

14

A patient with a hypodeveloped sacrum and fecal and urinary incontinence

CASSIE DO CARMO

CASE HISTORY

A 7-year-old female comes to your clinic with a history of caudal regression, absent sacrum, and fecal and urinary incontinence. The patient was previously adopted, so all of her medical history is unclear; however, adoption records show her only surgical history to include bilateral club foot repair and a ventricular peritoneal (VP) shunt. The mother reports that the patient is able to have voluntary bowel movements on the toilet, but wears pull-ups due to fecal smearing four to five times a week and daily urinary accidents. She has never been placed on a bowel regimen and is not currently taking any medications.

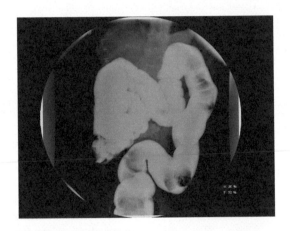

Figure 14.1 Contrast enema.

QUESTION 14.1

What is caudal regression syndrome?

Answer: Caudal regression syndrome refers to a constellation of anomalies resulting from a chromosomal insult in the early stages of gestation. There is a high association in infants of diabetic mothers. The spectrum of clinical presentation and the degree of caudal structural hypodevelopment correspond to the level of vertebral agenesis. Sphincter muscle and nerve innervation hypodevelopment can affect continence, thus in this population there is a higher incidence of fecal and urinary incontinence.

As a part of our evaluation, the patient had a contrast enema via her rectum with sacral imaging (Figures 14.1 and 14.2).

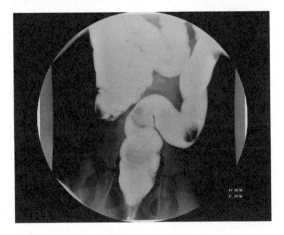

Figure 14.2 Contrast enema.

The post-evacuation film is shown in Figure 14.3. Sacral images are shown in Figures 14.4 through 14.7.

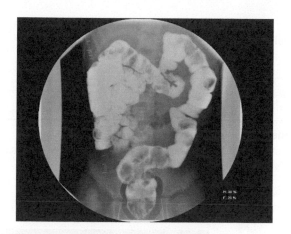

Figure 14.3 Post-evacuation film after contrast enema.

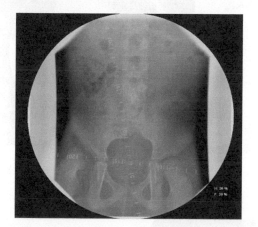

Figure 14.4 Anterior/posterior sacrum image.

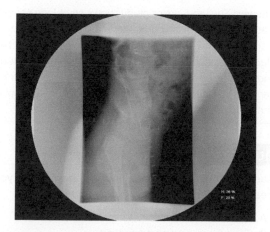

Figure 14.5 Lateral sacrum image.

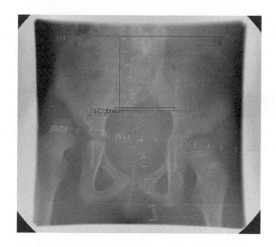

Figure 14.6 Anterior/posterior sacral ratio.

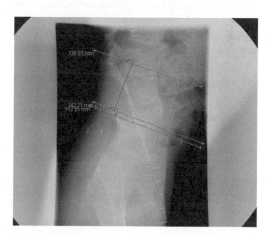

Figure 14.7 Lateral sacral ratio.

QUESTION 14.2

How do you interpret the findings on the contrast enema?

Answer: The contrast enema shows that there is a normal rectosigmoid ratio and a nondilated descending, transverse, and ascending colon. The patient's sacral ratio was measured in both the anterior/posterior view and lateral view: AP = 0.03 and LAT = 0.10. These findings are consistent with essentially an "absent" sacrum and caudal regression syndrome.

The patient had spinal magnetic resonance imaging (MRI) and its findings were consistent with caudal regression syndrome and showed no tethered cord. Her conus terminates at L1.

The patient's examination showed a normal anus as well as normal urinary and gynecological anatomy.

QUESTION 14.3

What would be the most valuable study to assess bladder function?

Answer: The patient had video urodynamics and a cystogram to assess her urologic system to try to explain her urinary incontinence (Figures 14.8 and 14.9).

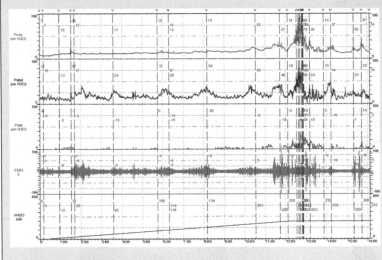

Figure 14.8 (See color insert.) Urodynamics tracing.

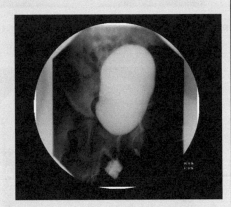

Figure 14.9 Cystogram image from video urodynamics.

The post-void image is shown in Figure 14.10.

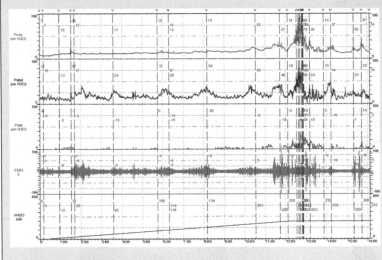

Figure 14.10 Post-void image from cystogram.

QUESTION 14.4

How do you interpret the urodynamics study?

Answer: The urodyamics study shows an oblong shaped bladder, with no vesicoureteral reflux, and a competent bladder neck. She has minimal trabeculation and her bladder capacity was 233 mL. Her post-void study shows retained urine of 175 mL, which is evidence of a neurogenic bladder. Overall, she has a safe bladder but is unable to completely empty.

QUESTION 14.5

Based on the urodynamics findings, how would you treat the patient's high post-void residual?

A. Clean intermittent catheterizations
B. Start the patient on oxybutynin

C. Instruct patient to do timed voiding and double voiding exercises

Answer: A. Clean intermittent catheterizations. Although the patient is able to urinate on her own and her urodynamic study showed a safe bladder, her high post-void residual is concerning. If the child continues to have a high post-void residual, this can contribute to vesicoureteral reflux, hydronephrosis, and urinary tract infections. The goal for clean intermittent catheterizations is to empty the bladder manually, lower its pressure, and thus keep the kidneys safe.

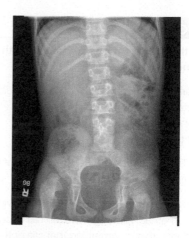

Figure 14.11 Abdominal X-ray 1 day after contrast enema.

QUESTION 14.6

Based on all of the testing discussed previously, what intervention do you think is appropriate for the patient's fecal incontinence?

A. Start the patient on a laxative program
B. Start the patient on an enema program

Answer: B. Due to the patient's poor sacrum and fecal incontinence, the patient would benefit from a mechanical program because we predict poor potential for voluntary bowel control.

QUESTION 14.7

What is your assessment of the X-ray in regard to stool volume?

Answer: There is stool throughout the colon. The goal is to have the descending colon and rectum clean of stool with large volume rectal enemas and this colon is not clean enough.

QUESTIONS 14.8

What changes would you make to this patient's regimen based on the X-ray and report?

A. Increase glycerin
B. Decrease glycerin
C. Increase saline
D. Decrease saline
E. Both A and C

Answer: The decision was made to increase the glycerin and saline (Answer E). The patient's X-ray showed stool throughout her colon and the patient reports two stool accidents within 24 hours of having the enema. This tells us that the patient not only needs an increased enema volume, but also needs the enema to be stronger, which can be accomplished by increasing the glycerin.

The patient was started on once a day enemas, which consisted of 400 mL of saline and 20 mL of glycerin with the goal of keeping her clean for a full 24 hours.

The patient's report of the 24 hours after the large volume enema along with the X-ray done after the enema are given in the following list.

Patient's report (Figure 14.11):

- Enema took 10 minutes to infuse
- Enema dwelled for 7 minutes
- Patient experienced mild cramping
- Patient had a large bowel movement on the toilet after the enema was completed
- She had two stool accidents 6 and 10 hours after the enema

The patient's regimen at the completion of the program was 450 mL of saline, 30 mL of glycerin, and 18 mL of baby soap. Fecal soiling improved, but she continued to have accidents once a week.

When returning for her 1-month bowel management follow-up appointment, the child's mother remains concerned about continued occasional fecal accidents and leaking during the enema. She continues to increase the amount of air in the balloon on the catheter and is currently inserting 70 mL of air into the balloon (max is 90 mL); despite this, it slips out regularly.

QUESTION 14.9

What further interventions do you think this patient could benefit from?

A. Continue rectal enemas with improved technique
B. Peristeen enemas
C. Malone appendicostomy
D. All of the above

Answer: The patient could benefit from all of the above (Answer D).

A. The patient has shown significant improvement on rectal enemas. Although she still has occasional accidents, this is something that can potentially be improved with regimen changes and better enema technique. The mother needs to pull back on the catheter so the balloon plugs the lumen at the anus to avoid leakage.

B. Peristeen is a great option for patients with spine and sacral anomalies. The balloon on the Peristeen system inflates to a much higher volume and contours better within the rectum than other catheters. Another benefit of using Peristeen is that no additives such as glycerin are needed due to the pressurized system.

C. Knowing that this patient benefits from a mechanical program, a Malone is a great long-term option. This is an intervention to consider if the patient is struggling with the rectal route. It also flushes the entire colon from the top down as opposed to just the descending colon, sigmoid, and rectum, which could help with the patient's occasional accidents and allow for more independence.

The patient has been doing well with clean intermittent catheterizations being performed three times a day. She is dry between catheterizations; however, the mother reports intermittent pain right above her pubic bone and is suspicious of bladder spasms.

QUESTION 14.10

What intervention is most appropriate to decrease the instance of bladder spasms?

A. Increase the frequency of the catheterizations
B. Start the patient on a bladder relaxant such as oxybutynin

C. Use over-the-counter analgesics like Ibuprofen or acetaminophen as needed

Answer: The answer is to start the patient on a medication such as oxybutynin to decrease bladder spasms (Answer B). Increasing the frequency of catheterizations can cause irritation to the bladder and thus bladder spasms can worsen. Over-the-counter analgesics can aid with mild pain; however, they will not stop smooth muscle, such as the bladder, from having spasms. The patient was started on 5 mg of oxybutynin twice a day.

KEY LEARNING POINTS

1. A patient with a poor spine/sacrum benefits from a mechanical program as opposed to an oral medication program to promote emptying of the colon.
2. A Malone and Peristeen are great options for patients with sacral anomalies because they allow for independence in performing the bowel regimen.
3. Ensure proper technique is being done when completing a flush. The goal is for the enema solution to infuse in 5–10 minutes. For rectal enemas, the solution should dwell for 5–10 minutes. During the infusion time and dwelling time with rectal enemas, it is important to make sure that the solution is not leaking. To stop or prevent leaking, the balloon on the catheter should be increased to 10 mL of air at a time until the leaking has stopped. Another technique to stop or prevent leaking is to pull on the catheter to create a seal between the balloon and the rectum. The patient should also be sitting on the toilet for 30 to 60 minutes after the enema to ensure that they have expelled all of the stool and solution. This will provide optimal results.

SUGGESTED READINGS

Midrio, P., Mosiello, G., Ausili, E. et al. 2016. Peristeen(®) transanal irrigation in paediatric patients with anorectal malformations and spinal cord lesions. *A Multicentre Italian Study*, 18(1), 86–93.

Wyndaele, J. J., Kovindha, A., Igawa, Y. et al. 2010. Neurologic fecal incontinence. *Neurourology and Urodynamics*, 29(1), 207–212.

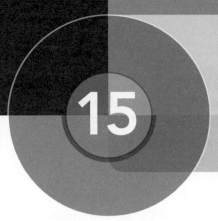

15

A patient with a spinal anomaly and fecal incontinence

CASSIE DO CARMO

CASE HISTORY

A 9-year-old patient comes to your clinic for his initial visit with a history of myelomeningocele, neurogenic bowel, and neurogenic bladder. The patient's past surgical history includes myelomeningocele closure. At another institution, to manage frequent impaction, a sigmoid resection and Malone appendicostomy were performed, and to manage urinary incontinence a colovesicostomy was done. The patient is currently doing a daily Malone flush which consists of 200 mL of saline and 10 mL of glycerin. His parents report that the flush infuses over 10 minutes and that the patient typically sits for 60 minutes.

They also report good output with the flush but with fecal soiling one to two times a day. She is dry, emptying her urinary stoma several times a day.

Fecal incontinence in patients with myelomeningocele is mainly due to abnormal recto-sigmoid compliance and recto-anal reflexes, loss of recto-anal sensitivity, and loss of voluntary control of the external anal sphincter. Constipation can be due to immobilization, abnormal colonic contractility, chronic sigmoid distention, and medications.

The patient had a contrast enema (Figures 15.1 and 15.2) and post-evacuation film (Figure 15.3).

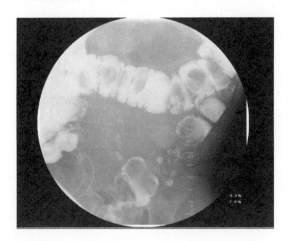

Figure 15.1 Contrast enema.

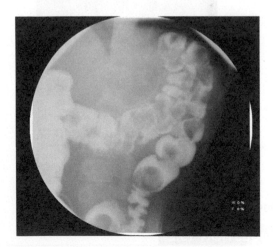

Figure 15.2 Contrast enema.

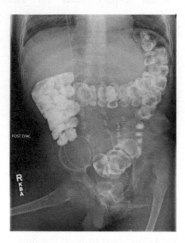

Figure 15.3 Post evacuation film after contrast enema.

QUESTION 15.1

How do you interpret the contrast study?

Answer: Non-dilated colon with normal haustra. Some of the sigmoid has been removed. The post-evacuation film shows residual contrast in the ascending and transverse colon. The left colon may be hyperperistaltic.

The patient had an abdominal X-ray taken on the day of their clinic visit, the day after the contrast enema (Figure 15.4).

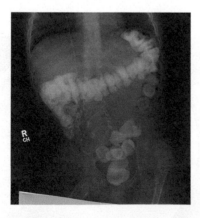

Figure 15.4 First bowel management X-ray.

QUESTION 15.2

How do you interpret the X-ray?

Answer: There is retained contrast throughout the colon with very small stool volume, consistent with slow motility.

QUESTION 15.3

Based on the patient's history and testing, how would you proceed with his bowel management plan?

  A. Attempt a laxative trial
  B. Continue current Malone flush regimen
  C. Continue Malone flushes, but with a stronger regimen

Answer: C. From the parent's report, he is having one to two episodes of fecal incontinence a day and his X-ray shows retained contrast and stool. These results tell us that the patient's current flush is not strong enough and therefore, he should be continued on Malone flushes but with an increased volume of 400 mL of saline and an increased stimulant using 20 mL of glycerin.

The patient's report and abdominal X-ray for the following day is given.

  Patient's report:

- Flush took 14 minutes to infuse
- Sat on the toilet for 50 minutes
- No symptoms
- No accidents

QUESTION 15.4

How do you interpret the abdominal X-ray (Figure 15.5)?

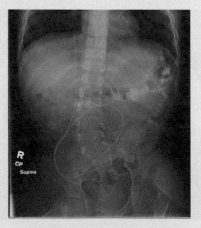

Figure 15.5 Second bowel management X-ray.

Answer: There is stool accumulation in the right side of the colon.

QUESTION 15.5

Based on the patient's report and abdominal X-ray, what changes would you make to the flush?

A. Increase glycerin
B. Decrease glycerin
C. Add Castile soap
D. Decrease saline

Answer: The answer is increase the glycerin (Answer A). The X-ray showed increased stool accumulation in comparison to the previous X-ray. The mother reports he is asymptomatic and not having accidents. Increasing the glycerin will make the flush stronger to ensure the entire colon is being cleaned out to prevent potential leakage between flushes.

The patient was placed on a Malone flush of 400 mL of saline and now 30 mL of glycerin. This regimen remained the same throughout the rest of the bowel management program and he remained clean between flushes.

The patient returned to clinic for his 1 month follow-up appointment. His mother reports that he continues to do well on his current flush of 400 mL of saline and 30 mL of glycerin with no symptoms and no accidents.

An X-ray was taken 17 hours after flush was completed (Figure 15.6).

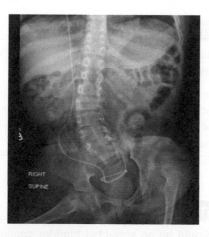

Figure 15.6 One month follow up X-ray for bowel management.

QUESTION 15.6

How do you interpret this X-ray?

Answer: There is some stool in the ascending and transverse colon. The descending colon and rectum are clean.

QUESTION 15.7

Based on the patient's report and abdominal X-ray, what would you recommend?

A. Increase glycerin
B. Decrease glycerin
C. Add Castile
D. Keep regimen the same

Answer: The answer is to keep the regimen the same (Answer D). Although the patient's abdominal X-ray shows stool in the ascending and transverse colon, the X-ray was taken 17 hours after the flush was completed. It is to be expected to have some stool accumulation during that time. The patient's report guides you in this situation. You can also have the patient repeat the X-ray within 2 hours of the flush being completed to ensure the flush is adequate.

KEY LEARNING POINTS

1. An abdominal X-ray and the patient report are both important and necessary when determining a regimen change.
2. Timing of the flush in relation to the X-ray is vital in obtaining accurate results. If a patient obtains an abdominal X-ray 20 hours after their enema/ antegrade enema, this will show us inaccurate data about how well the regimen is working as enough time has passed for stool to move within the colon. It is best to obtain an X-ray as soon after the flush as possible to provide the most accurate assessment of how well the regimen is working to clean the colon.
3. Antegrade options for patients with spinal anomalies not only aid with fecal incontinence but provide for more independence. With a Malone the patient is able to do the flush on their own and can gain more confidence in their social life, such as attending sleepovers at a friend's house.

SUGGESTED READING

Krogh, K. & Christensen, P. 2009. Neurogenic colorectal and pelvic floor dysfunction. *Best Practice & Research: Clinical Gastroenterology*, 23, 531–543.

16

A pediatric patient with spina bifida in need of a urological reconstruction

CHERYL BAXTER

CASE HISTORY

An 8-year-old female with a low lumbar myelomeningocele and paraplegia presents to your clinic for assistance with bowel management because of her daily soiling. Her pertinent past surgical history

includes a ventricular peritoneal shunt, vesicostomy that was closed at age 5 years at which point she underwent an appendicovesicostomy (Mitrofanoff), bladder augmentation, and cecostomy. No bladder neck tightening or closure was performed. Within a few months of placement of the Mitrofanoff, the stoma closed at the skin level and was no longer accessible. She is leaking urine constantly from her urethra. Her mother has attempted clean intermittent catheterization every 3 hours in an effort to keep her dry, but this was not successful.

QUESTION 16.1

With regards to her bladder status, what testing would you like to see at this point to help you figure out her optimal management?

Answer: Videourodynamic evaluation would be indicated (Figure 16.1).

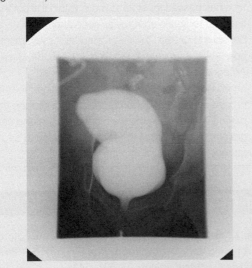

Figure 16.1 Videourodynamic image with open bladder neck.

QUESTION 16.2

How do you interpret the findings on the voiding cystourethrogram?

Answer: The voiding cystourethrogram (VCUG) shows a smooth contour of the bladder. The irregularity of the superior lateral aspect of the bladder demonstrates the prior bladder augmentation.

QUESTION 16.3

What would be an expected bladder capacity in a 8-year-old child?

Answer: Utilizing the Koff formula of (age (years) + 2) × 30 = bladder capacity in mL (Figure 16.2):

$$8 + 2 = 10 \times 30 = 300 \text{ mL}$$

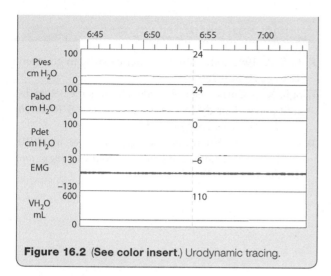

Figure 16.2 **(See color insert.)** Urodynamic tracing.

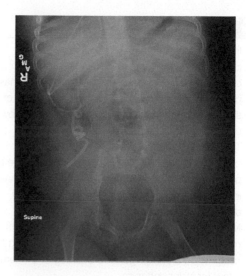

Figure 16.3 Abdominal radiograph.

The VCUG showed a leak at 172 mL with a pressure of 10 cm H_2O and no vesicouretheral reflux.

QUESTION 16.4

What are the indicators of poor urethral outlet resistance in this patient?

Answer: The indicators of poor urethral outlet resistance are low pressures (less than 40 cm H_2O) with leakage of urine at less than expected bladder capacity. Additionally, the bladder neck can be seen open on images during a VCUG (see Figure 16.1). In this patient, the leakage at low bladder pressures allow the patient's bladder to maintain a low-pressure reservoir, which assists in protecting the upper tract renal system. However, bladder neck incompetence leads to persistent urinary incontinence despite clean intermittent catheterization on a timed basis. In order for her to achieve urinary continence, she would require a bladder neck reconstruction.

QUESTION 16.5

How do you interpret this X-ray?

Answer: The X-ray shows no stool in her rectum but there is stool accumulation in the descending colon. She has a Chait™ cecostomy tube in her right lower quadrant.

QUESTION 16.6

What changes in her bowel flush regimen would you change based on the history and evaluation of the abdominal X-ray done two hours following a flush?

Answer: She is having stool incontinence 12 hours after her flush. Increasing the strength of her flush by increasing her glycerin to 30 mL may help to move the remaining stool from her descending colon.

The current bowel regimen is 400 mL of normal saline and 20 mL of glycerin via the cecostomy tube daily. She is having daily soiling accidents. Her flush is completed between 7 and 8 P.M. and her accidents occur upon waking (Figure 16.3).

At this time, her family is considering a redo of her Mitrofanoff channel to open it and a bladder neck reconstruction to achieve urinary continence. Strengthening her flush allowed her to remain clean between flushes.

KEY LEARNING POINTS

1. In the past two decades, the number of interventions available to individuals with neurogenic bladder and bowel as a result of spina bifida has grown tremendously. As a result, the number of surgical interventions aimed at bladder and bowel continence have increased dramatically.

2. The goals of management of a neurogenic bladder in patients with myelomeningocele are to preserve renal function and have the patient have independent continence at a developmentally appropriate age.

3. Many patients with spina bifida have slow colonic motility and laxity of the anal sphincter making fecal continence a challenge. Use of antegrade enemas allow for independence.

4. Patients with spina bifida have poor outlet resistance leading to chronic urinary incontinence. Bladder neck reconstruction can add resistance to improve urinary continence.

5. Ideally, good bowel management should be in place prior to the urological reconstruction. It can improve urinary continence in some patients. Knowing the amount and time needed to flush a colon can help the surgeon decide if some sigmoid colon should be removed to help make the flush more efficient. This is particularly useful in a case where the sigmoid could be used to perform a bladder augmentation (Figure 16.4).

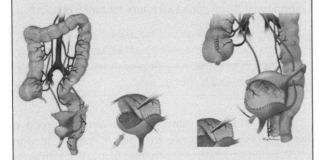

Figure 16.4 Use of sigmoid colon to augment the bladder.

SUGGESTED READINGS

Koff, S. A. 1983. Estimating bladder capacity in children. *Urology*, 1, 248–250.

Krogh, K. & Christensen, P. 2009. Neurogenic colorectal and pelvic floor dysfunction. *Best Practice & Research: Clinical Gastroenterology*, 23, 531–543.

Wyndaele, J. J., Kovindha, A., Igawa, Y. et al. 2010. Neurologic fecal incontinence. *Neurourology and Urodynamics*, 29(1), 207–212.

17

A young adult with quadriplegia and fecal incontinence due to spinal cord injury (SCI)

CHERYL BAXTER

A 24-year-old female has a history of leukemia and quadriplegia secondary to intrathecal injection of chemotherapy. Her surgical history includes a Monti channel (using a segment of small bowel) for antegrade colonic flushes (with a Chait™ tube in it) and an appendicovesicostomy (mitrofanoff) catheterizable channel for urine.

She is currently struggling with her antegrade flushes. She reports pain and vomiting with her flushes of 400 mL of saline and 20 mL of glycerin. She is having intermittent stool accidents several times per week.

She is doing well from a urinary standpoint on clean intermittent catheterizations of the appendicovesicostomy.

A contrast enema was completed for an initial evaluation (Figures 17.1 and 17.2).

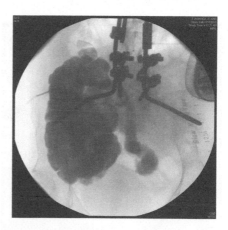

Figure 17.2 Contrast enema, a post-evacuation image.

QUESTION 17.1

What is your interpretation of this image of the contrast enema?

Answer: Contrast initially fills the terminal ileum and then fills the cecum, with significant retrograde flow of contrast into small bowel.

QUESTION 17.2

What is the significance of contrast refluxing back into the small bowel?

Answer: The ileocecal (IC) valve is incompetent in some patients and the instillation of a flush regimen can lead to symptoms of nausea and vomiting, pain with flush, and prolonged sit times for evacuation. Of course, the flush itself is not entering the colon and therefore the patient will not successfully evacuate.

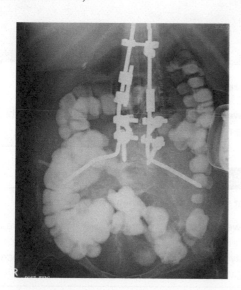

Figure 17.1 Contrast enema.

QUESTION 17.3

What treatment options would be the best approach?

A. Increase the volume and strength of the flush
B. Ask the patient to lie on their left side to facilitate closure of IC valve prior to flush
C. Have interventional radiology place a threaded tube (such as a jejunal tube) through the cecostomy to the mid-right colon
D. Administer ondansetron 4 mg 1 hour prior to flush

Answer: C is the correct answer. Facilitation of the flush into the right colon may reduce the incidence of IC reflux and the associated symptoms (Figure 17.3).

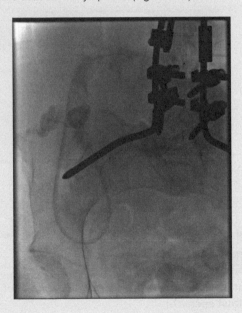

Figure 17.3 Fluoroscopic image of J-tube placed in antegrade channel.

The image shows a successful placement of a 45 cm length tube with a 3.5 cm stem length. The fluoroscopic image shows the end of the tube in the right transverse colon.

Her antegrade flushes were changed to 500 mL of saline and 30 mL of glycerin once per day. Her symptoms resolved with the placement of the threaded tube into the right colon, and she remained clean.

Five months after placement of the tube, she began to experience minimal output with flushes.

QUESTION 17.4

What would be the next step in the management of this patient?

A. Increase the glycerin to 35 mL
B. Increase the volume of the saline
C. Obtain an X-ray 2 hours after a flush to determine stool burden
D. All of the above

Answer: C. Rationale—an X-ray can provide you with the current stool burden to determine if there are changes needed for the flush. Inquire as to changes in diet, fluid intake, and activity occurring within 24 hours of the problematic flush.

QUESTION 17.5

How do you interpret this X-ray (Figure 17.4)?

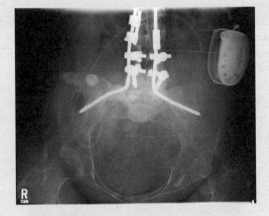

Figure 17.4 Abdominal X-ray.

Answer: The X-ray shows an increase in the stool burden in the rectum.

QUESTION 17.6

What would you recommend now?

Answer: Increasing the strength of the flush by increasing glycerin or adding Castile soap can result in improved emptying of stool. The recommendation was to increase the glycerin to 35 mL.

The follow-up abdominal X-ray (Figure 17.5) was done 1 week after increasing the glycerin to 35 mL with 400 mL of saline, the X-ray was clean and she is clean as well with no symptoms associated with the flush.

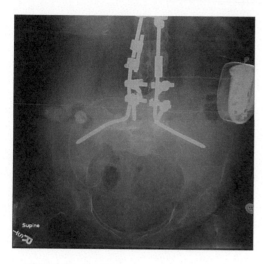

Figure 17.5 Abdominal X-ray.

KEY LEARNING POINTS

1. In patients with spinal cord injury (SCI), both upper motor neuron injury or dysfunction and lower motor neuron damage can be present depending on the level of the injury. Upper motor injury results in a hyperreflexic bowel with increased rectal and sigmoid compliance as well as increased anal sphincter tone, thus promoting stool retention and constipation. Lower motor neuron damage results in areflexic bowel, loss of peristalsis with resultant slower stool propulsion, reduced rectal compliance, and lax anal tone. These factors contribute to both constipation and fecal incontinence.

2. Bowel dysfunction caused by lower neuron SCI can lead to slow transit times, decreased sphincter tone, and constipation with fecal incontinence. Therefore, to get such a patient clean, the treatment required is a mechanical regimen.
3. Ileocecal valve reflux can lead to nausea, vomiting, and abdominal pain. This can lead to an unsuccessful flush that does not get to the colon.
4. Correct positioning of the antegrade catheter by an interventional radiologist can lead to improvement in the flushes.
5. Problematic flushes require a contrast study via the Malone or cecostomy to simulate the flush to try to understand why the symptoms are occurring.

SUGGESTED READINGS

Krassioukov, A., Eng, J. J., Claxton, G., Sakakibara, B. M., & Shum, S. 2010. Neurogenic bowel management after spinal cord injury: A systematic review of the evidence. *Spinal Cord*, 48(10), 718–733.

Krogh, K. & Christensen, P. 2009. Neurogenic colorectal and pelvic floor dysfunction. *Best Practice & Research: Clinical Gastroenterolog*, 23, 531–543.

			POINTS
ARM TYPE	Perineal Fistula	1	
	Rectal Stenosis	1	
	Rectal Atresia	1	
	Rectovestibular Fistula	1	
	Rectobulbar Fistula	1	
	Imperforate Anus Without Fistula	1	
	Cloaca < 3 cm Common Channel	2	
	Rectoprostatic Fistula	2	
	Rectovaginal Fistula	2	
	Recto–bladder neck Fistula	3	
	Cloaca > 3 cm Common Channel	3	
	Cloacal Exstrophy	3	

SPINE	Normal Termination of the Conus (L1–L2)	1
	Normal Filum Appearance	1
	Abnormally Low Termination of the Conus (Below L3)	2
	Abnormal Fatty Thickening of Filum	2
	Myelomeningocele	3

SACRUM	Sacral Ratio = Greater than 0.7	1
	Sacral Ratio = Between 0.4 and 0.69	2
	Hemisacrum	2
	Sacral Hemivertebrae	2
	Presacral Mass	2
	Sacral Ratio = Less than 0.4	3

TOTAL POINTS

3–4 = Good
Potential for continence

5–6 = Fair
Potential for continence

7–9 = Poor
Potential for continence

Figure II.1 ARM Index.

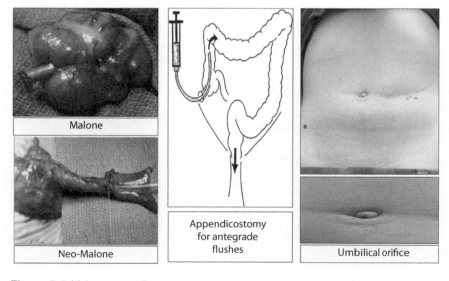

Malone

Neo-Malone

Appendicostomy for antegrade flushes

Umbilical orifice

Figure 5.4 Malone appendicostomy.

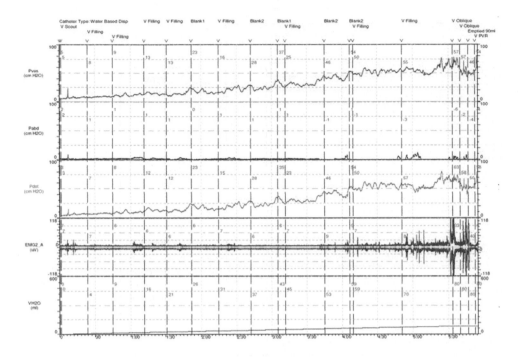

Figure 6.3 Urodynamics.

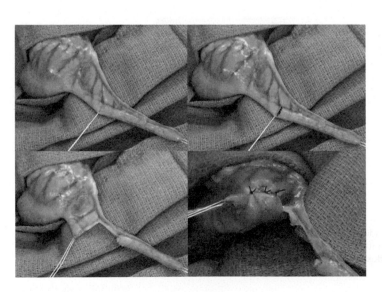

Figure 6.4 Split Malone appendicostomy.

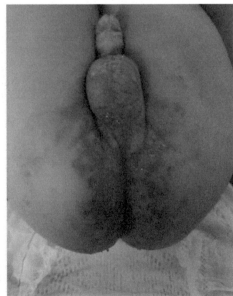

Figure 12.3 Perineum.

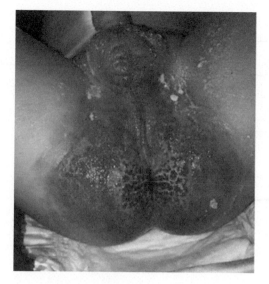

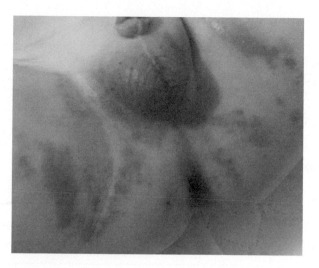

Figure 12.6 Perineum.

Figure 12.4 Perineum.

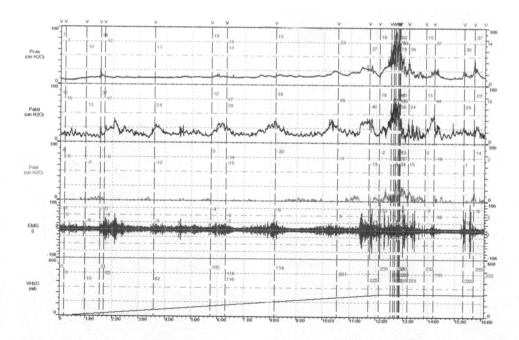

Figure 14.8 Urodynamics tracing.

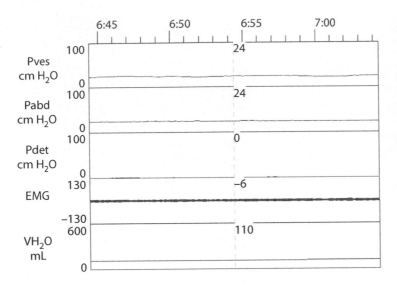

Figure 16.2 Urodynamic tracing.

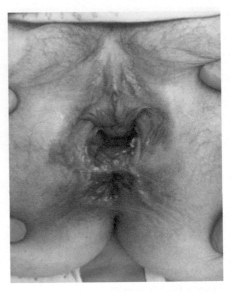

Figure 29.4 EUA image of a disrupted perineal body.

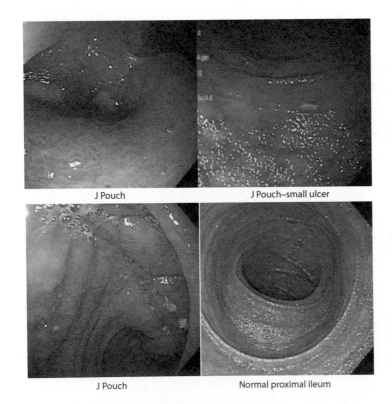

J Pouch

J Pouch–small ulcer

J Pouch

Normal proximal ileum

Figure 31.1 Pouchoscopy images.

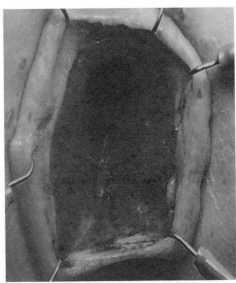

Figure 34.1 EUA showing a last dentate line.

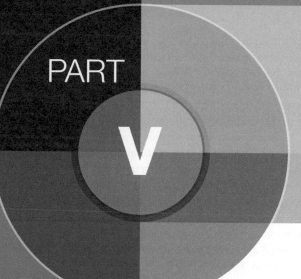

PART V

FUNCTIONAL CONSTIPATION

INTRODUCTION

Meghan Fisher

Functional or idiopathic constipation is defined as the inability to effectively evacuate stool from the colon on a daily basis with no underlying congenital surgical condition. It is a very common problem in pediatrics. Although many patients do not have an underlying medical disease, some may have anomalies within the colon, sphincter, or have behavioral issues that make the constipation difficult to manage. Common symptoms include abdominal pain, bloating, distension, and poor appetite. Some patients also experience fecal incontinence owing to overflow of stool or fecal impaction. A typical case of fecal impaction with soiling will be discussed in this section. Overall, these patients have good potential for bowel control as they have normal anatomy, sphincters, and spinal/sacral anatomy. Patients with a mild form of the disease can be managed with stool softeners or behavioral therapy, while the more severe cases may require intensive bowel management treatment, botulinum toxin injections into the anal canal, or surgery (antegrade access for enemas, colonic resection). These interventions will be reviewed within this section, including cases of failure of cecostomy flushes and rectal enemas, and poor emptying despite a colonic resection.

This disease process can appear at many different times in a patient's life. In early childhood, painful stools can cause fear of having a bowel movement. Children dread repeating the experience and begin to intentionally avoid having bowel movements. Delayed treatment can result in withholding behavior, which can lead to worsening constipation. A patient who had severe withholding or internal sphincter achalasia will be described. Changes in stool patterns and consistency occur after the introduction of solids, at time of toilet training, and the starting of school. When any of these symptoms or patterns are observed, it is important to involve a medical team. An evaluation by a pediatric gastroenterologist helps to rule other known causes of constipation including Hirschsprung disease, celiac disease, thyroid problems, food allergies, and cystic fibrosis. They can also begin the patient on a bowel regimen.

If multiple therapies have been attempted, yet the patient's constipation does not improve, escalation to a motility/colorectal specialist should be initiated. Upon initial evaluation, a medical history should be obtained, including the patient's current bowel routine, previous failed regimens, soiling history, and developmental status. A contrast study allows evaluation of the colonic anatomy, particularly noting any redundancy and/or dilation. After consideration of these items, the patient can be started on either a rectal enema regimen or stimulant laxative with water-soluble fiber. If a flush or laxative program has been maximized and the patient has still not achieved the goal of effective evacuation without accidents, other options must be considered. Failure of medical management in these patients also includes continued constipation despite treatment, persistent soiling, and/or intolerance of medications due to side effects.

Additionally, there are patients who do not follow the traditional pattern of constipation. An example of this would be a patient who is failing to thrive, has symptoms of severe abdominal distension or straining to stool, yet has a rectal biopsy that is negative for Hirschsprung disease. Such a patient requires motility testing and potentially a diversion of stool with an ileostomy, a unique challenge to colorectal and motility teams, and described as a case in this section (Figure 1).

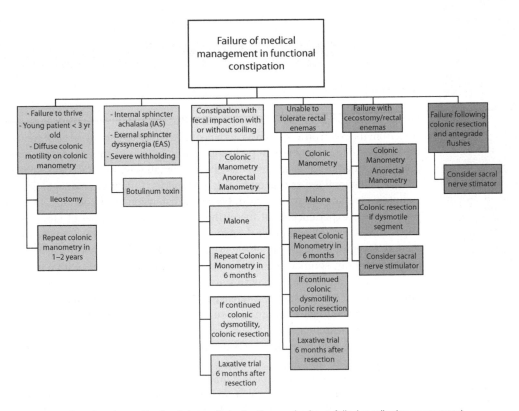

Figure 1 Functional constipation interventions for those who have failed medical management.

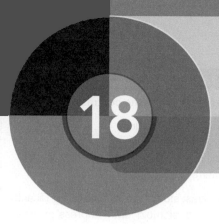

A case of diffuse colonic dysmotility

18

SARAH DRIESBACH

A 4-year-old female with a history of chronic constipation since 3 months of age presents to your clinic. She has remained at the bottom of her growth curve and has a diagnosis of failure to thrive. Her urologist had referred her to a gastroenterologist after finding a large fecal impaction during a renal ultrasound that was felt to be causing urinary retention. Despite multiple laxative regimens implemented, as well as daily enemas and in-patient disimpactions, she is unable to reliably empty her colon and was referred to the colorectal surgery clinic for consideration of surgical options.

INITIAL EVALUATION

QUESTION 18.1

What are your potential differential diagnoses for a patient with persistent constipation and failure to thrive despite multiple modalities of medical therapy? What data will you need to rule out or confirm each one?

DIFFERENTIAL DIAGNOSES

HIRSCHSPRUNG DISEASE

Given this history, evaluation for Hirschsprung disease (HD) is warranted. A biopsy was performed and showed no ganglion cells, which was highly suggestive of HD, but squamous epithelium was noted in the specimen. Findings that would support a diagnosis of HD would include the absence of ganglion cells, the presence of hypertrophic nerves, and decreased or absent calretinin-immunoreactive fibers in the lamina propria on calretinin staining. However, this patient's nerves were of normal size and her calretinin staining was normal. When this scenario occurs, the clinician should be suspicious that the biopsy was taken too low, in the normally aganglionic region of the anal canal. This is consistent with the findings of squamous epithelium on the pathology report; thus, this is an inadequate evaluation for HD.

ANORECTAL MALFORMATION

Exam of this patient's perineum and anus under anesthesia at the time of the biopsy revealed a well-centered anus that is a size 18 Hegar. These findings are normal and not concerning for any type of anorectal malformation.

MOTILITY DISORDER

This patient's contrast study is pictured in Figures 18.1 through 18.3:

- Lateral view of rectum (Figure 18.1)
- AP view of rectum (Figure 18.2)
- Post-evacuation view (Figure 18.3)

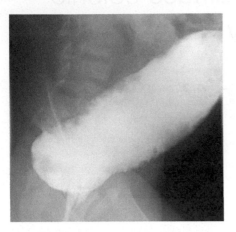

Figure 18.1 Contrast study lateral view of rectum.

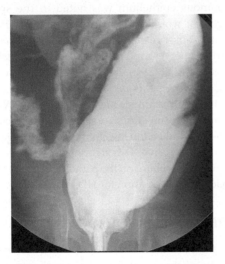

Figure 18.2 Contrast study AP view of rectum.

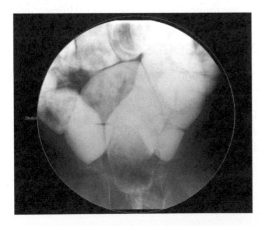

Figure 18.3 Contrast study post evacuation view.

QUESTION 18.2

What is your assessment of the contrast study?

A. Normal rectum, normal colon
B. Dilated rectum, dilated colon
C. Normal rectum, dilated colon
D. Dilated rectum, normal colon

Answer: The contrast study demonstrates a significantly dilated rectum and sigmoid with impressive post-evacuation residual contrast (Answer B). It should also be noted that there are only very few haustra throughout the colon, indicating poor peristalsis.

QUESTION 18.3

If the lateral view of this patient's contrast study had showed a widened presacral space, what might you suspect to be the cause of her constipation and what additional testing would you order?

Answer: Quite rare, but important to think about, presacral masses can encroach upon the rectosigmoid colon and obstruct the flow of stool, causing constipation. A presacral mass can be detected on the lateral views of a contrast study, which would present as a widened presacral space. If this finding was evident, the next step would be to obtain an MRI of the pelvis to evaluate for a presacral mass.

QUESTION 18.4

What would you do next?

Answer: This patient's refractory constipation (failure of medical management) and contrast study showing evidence of chronic colonic dilation and poor motility prompted anorectal and colonic motility testing. This patient's anorectal manometry (AMAN) was normal, with a positive rectoanal inhibitory reflex (RAIR), a normal resting pressure, and an effective push and squeeze. However, her colonic manometry (CMAN) showed total colonic dysmotility, no high amplitude propagating contractions even with stimulants, and a possible neurogenic pattern to her dysmotility.

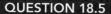

QUESTION 18.5

The rectal biopsy was potentially suspicious for HD. Based on the additional testing that has been obtained, can we safely exclude HD as a possible diagnosis?

Answer: Yes, HD can definitely be ruled out based on the anorectal manometry study. Children with HD do not have a RAIR, therefore a finding of a positive RAIR on AMAN testing excludes HD as a possible diagnosis. With the rectal biopsy showing no ganglion cells and no hypertrophic nerves in a patient who has a positive RAIR, we already suspected that the biopsy was taken too low.

QUESTION 18.6

What other testing do these results make you consider?

- A. Magnetic resonance imaging of the lumbar spine and pelvis
- B. Colonoscopy
- C. Rigid sigmoidoscopy
- D. Upper GI motility testing

Spinal anomalies/presacral mass
This patient's refractory constipation and possible neurogenic component to the dysmotility found on her CMAN indicate that spinal anomalies including spina bifida occulta, tethered cord, and spinal tumor need to be considered (Answer A). However, MRI testing of the lumbar spine was normal.

MANAGEMENT

QUESTION 18.7

What are your main goals in treating this patient? What are your main concerns?

Answer: Our primary concerns were the patient's failure to thrive and her inability to empty her colon despite maximal medical therapy. Her total colonic dysmotility was the primary cause of both problems. Our goal was to give the patient a way to consistently empty her bowels in order to facilitate growth and prevent fecal impaction.

QUESTION 18.8

What intervention would you recommend?

Answer: The patient underwent an ileostomy to allow the bowel to rest and to improve her nutritional status. A repeat rectal biopsy and colonic biopsies were also performed so we could be absolutely certain that this was not a case of total colonic Hirschsprung disease. All biopsy results were normal. A mucous fistula was also created to provide an outlet for the patient's intestinal secretions as well as a Malone appendicostomy to allow for future antegrade flushes of the colon once the ileostomy is closed and for repeat motility testing via an antegrade route. In the future, antegrade flushes will be the best choice for this patient, because they can mechanically empty the entire colon compared to just the rectum and descending colon with rectal enemas. It is likely that this will need to be done in conjunction with a colonic resection. Antegrade flushes are more likely to be successful than rectal enemas in a patient with total colonic dysmotility, as rectal enemas may still allow for stool accumulation proximal to the area that can be reached rectally. A Malone alone for antegrade enemas could also be considered, but likely will not be effective at emptying the colon without a resection, given her diffuse dysmotility.

QUESTION 18.9

What if this patient's clinical picture had been the same, but without failure to thrive?

Answer: If this patient had not had growth concerns, a Malone appendicostomy may have been sufficient to allow her to empty her colon consistently with antegrade flushes. It is the failure to thrive that pushed us to intervene with an ileostomy as a first step to break the cycle of constipation and worsening failure to thrive.

Following the ileostomy, this patient had consistently good stool output. Her growth improved and she continued to thrive for months following surgery (Figures 18.4 and 18.5).

At 8 months postop, she was admitted for severe abdominal pain. The X-ray shown in Figure 18.6 was obtained.

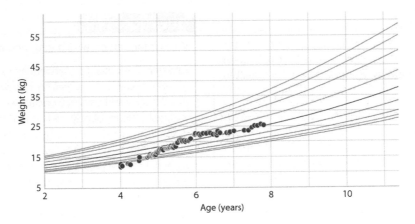

Figure 18.4 Growth curve for weight.

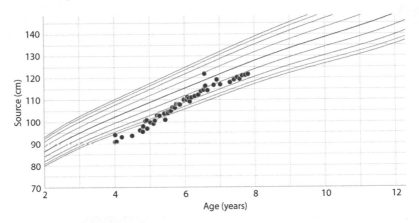

Figure 18.5 Growth curve for height.

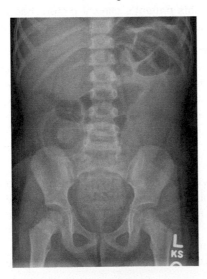

Figure 18.6 Eight month postop X-ray.

QUESTION 18.10

What does this X-ray show?

Answer: Despite being diverted with an ileostomy, she had developed a large fecal impaction of accumulated mucous in her rectum.

QUESTION 18.11

How did a diverted patient develop such a large fecal impaction? How could we have prevented this?

Answer: Despite being diverted, this patient's severe dysmotility caused an impaction to develop due to ongoing mucus production in the colon and the colon's inability to pass the mucous. Our treatment was an in-patient bowel cleanout via the Malone appendicostomy to remove the impaction followed by weekly antegrade colonic flushes at home to keep her diverted colon clean. This accumulation could have been prevented by having the patient perform intermittent antegrade flushes via the Malone appendicostomy starting immediately following the ileostomy.

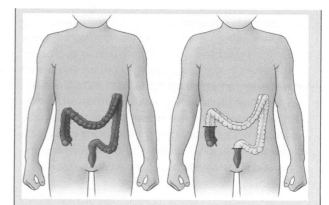

Figure 18.7 Extended resection.

QUESTION 18.12

What is your plan for this patient moving forward?

Answer: Our long-term plan for this patient was to retest her colon's motility after a period of colonic diversion to see if it regained any function. Repeat CMAN through the Malone appendicostomy site one year postop still showed myopathic dysmotility present throughout her colon, no activity at baseline or postprandial phase, low amplitude propagating contractions (LAPCs) with two separate stimulants, and patient was symptomatic, but no high amplitude propagating contractions (HAPCs).

QUESTION 18.13

What is the next step for a patient with diffuse colonic dysmotility with no improvement in colonic function after initial treatment with an ileostomy?

- A. Ileostomy long term
- B. Colectomy, derotation of colon, plication of appendicostomy
- C. Close ileostomy, start Malone flushes daily
- D. Close ileostomy, perform end colostomy

Answer: How to handle such a rare scenario is unclear. We chose to perform an ileostomy closure and an extended colectomy with preservation and derotation of the right colon with a right colon to rectum anastomosis, similar to the Deloyer's procedure done in adults (see Figures 18.7 through 18.9) (Manceau et al., 2012) (Answer B). We also chose to empirically inject botulinum toxin into the anal canal. The botulinum toxin injection was added to her surgery based on the previous AMAN findings of a high resting pressure, which suggests some degree of difficulty with the sphincters' ability to relax. Botulinum

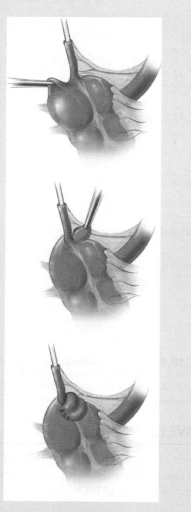

Figure 18.8 Malone appendicosotmy.

toxin promotes relaxation of the internal and external anal sphincters, which can in turn facilitate colonic emptying. The Malone was taken down from the umbilicus, plicated, and replaced. In the postoperative period, she was started on twice daily small Malone flushes with 150 mL of saline and 10 mL of glycerin, and a constipating diet to help form solid stool. Doing two smaller volume flushes in the immediate postoperative period will allow the colon to be adequately flushed while avoiding over-distending the bowel and potentially damaging the anastomoses.

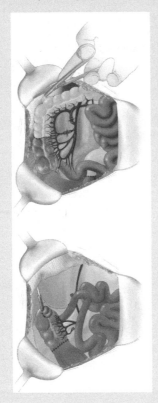

Figure 18.9 Extended resection, derotation of right colon, right colon to rectum anastomosis. (Adapted from Manceau, G. et al. 2012. *Diseases of the Colon & Rectum*, 55(3): 363–368.)

TWO WEEK POSTOP VISIT

The patient is tolerating flushes well but still having stools between flushes three times per week. A follow-up X-ray was obtained (Figure 18.10).

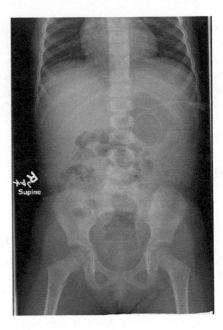

Figure 18.10 Two week postop X-ray.

QUESTION 18.14

What is your assessment of this X-ray?

Answer: The X-ray shows a clean rectum and colon. Our plan was to continue Malone flushes twice daily with 150 mL of saline and 10 mL of glycerin.

ONE MONTH POSTOPERATIVE VISIT

The patient is tolerating flushes, still stooling three times per week between flushes, and is otherwise clean. The patient found the catheterization of the Malone channel to be uncomfortable, so her parents chose to have a Chait tube placed into her Malone site to allow for easier access to the colon without having to catheterize. The Chait tube is visible on the X-ray shown in Figure 18.11.

- Clean rectum and colon
- *Plan*: Malone flushes with 300 mL of saline and 20 mL of glycerin

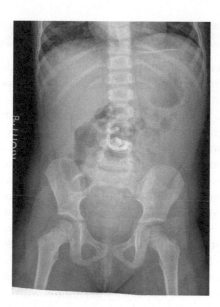

Figure 18.11 One month postop X-ray.

THREE MONTH POSTOPERATIVE VISIT

The patient reports a sit time during the flush of 1 hour and decreased stool output. She reports no accidents, but does report abdominal pain. A follow-up X-ray was obtained (Figure 18.12).

QUESTION 18.15

What does this X-ray show?

A. Clean X-ray
B. Increased stool throughout
C. Increased stool in the rectum and right colon
D. Increased stool in the right colon only

Answer: The X-ray shows increased stool in the rectum and right colon (Answer C). Our plan was to do two flushes 2 hours apart for a cleanout, increase the strength of the flush to 300 mL of saline with 30 mL of glycerin, and repeat botulinum toxin injection to the anal canal based on the patient's increased difficulty clearing stool. We know that botulinum toxin wears off after approximately 3 months, and this patient had an increase in obstructive symptoms about 3 months following her last botulinum toxin injection.

ONE WEEK FOLLOW-UP

The patient reported no accidents and has had a small amount of voluntary liquid stool between flushes two to three times since the regimen change. A follow-up X-ray was obtained and is pictured (Figure 18.13).

This patient's X-ray is clean and much improved compared to the previous X-ray.

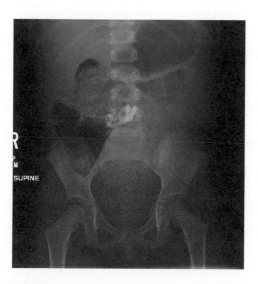

Figure 18.12 Three month postop X-ray.

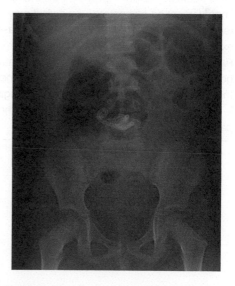

Figure 18.13 X-ray 1 week after regimen increase.

QUESTION 18.16

What is your follow-up plan?

A. Continue flushes once daily with 300 mL saline and 30 mL glycerin

B. Decrease flushes to 300 mL saline and 10 mL glycerin

C. Increase the strength of the flush to 300 mL saline, 30 mL glycerin, and 9 mL Castile soap

D. Stop flushes and start rectal enemas with 300 mL saline only

Answer: Continue flushes once daily with 300 mL saline and 30 mL glycerin, as the patient is clean and doing well (Answer A).

KEY LEARNING POINTS

1. Motility testing is a crucial step when a patient has intractable constipation despite optimal medical therapy.
2. Patients with diffuse colonic dysmotility are at high risk for failure to thrive, and may require an ileostomy to allow for proper growth.
3. Repeat colonic manometry testing is necessary after a period of bowel rest with an ileostomy. Often, colonic motility improves. If there is no improvement on manometry, the patient may require further surgical intervention, in this case an extended colonic resection.
4. Patients with diffuse colonic dysmotility still have good potential to be socially clean and continent in the future, therefore titration of their bowel regimen is necessary until X-rays are clean and until the patient is free from accidents.

SUGGESTED READINGS

Di Lorenzo, C. 2001. Pediatric anorectal disorders. *Gastroenterology Clinics of North America*, 30(1), 269–87.

Husain, S. & Di Lorenzo, C. 2002. Motility disorders. Diagnosis and treatment for the pediatric patient. *Pediatric Clinics of North America*, 49(1), 27–51.

Manceau, G., Karoui, M., Breton, S., Blanchet, A., Rousseau, G., Savier, E., Siksik, J., Vaillant, J., & Hannoun, L. 2012. Right colon to rectal anastomosis (Deloyers procedure) as a salvage technique for low colorectal or coloanal anastomosis: Postoperative and long-term outcomes. *Diseases of the Colon & Rectum*, 55(3), 363–368.

Pensabene, L., Youssef, N., Griffiths, J. & Di Lorenzo, C. 2003. Colonic manometry in children with defecatory disorders. Role in diagnosis and management. *The American Journal of Gastroenterology* 98(5), 1052–1057.

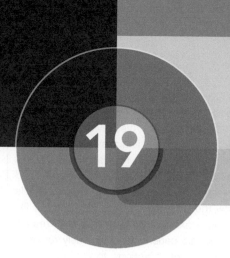

A patient with chronic constipation and sphincter dysfunction

SARAH DRIESBACH

19

CASE HISTORY

A 2-year-old male with a history of chronic constipation since 1 year of age with failure to thrive presents to your clinic. Initially, his providers thought he had Hirschsprung disease (HD.) His contrast study was thought to be suspicious for this disease, but a full thickness rectal biopsy revealed ganglion cells and no hypertrophic nerves. Treatment prior to presenting to us included high doses of various stimulant laxatives, rectal irrigations, and three separate anal botulinum toxin injections with no significant improvement. The patient had a previous myectomy performed as well, which improved his symptoms temporarily but did not resolve them. His contrast study can be seen in Figures 19.1 and 19.2.

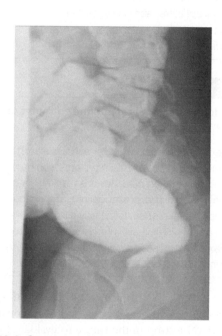

Figure 19.2 Contrast study, lateral view.

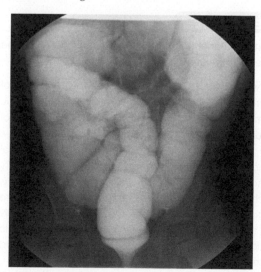

Figure 19.1 Contrast study, AP view.

QUESTION 19.1

What is your interpretation of the contrast study?

Answer: The contrast study showed a redundant, dilated colon as well as a dilated rectosigmoid with reverse rectosigmoid ratio on both AP and lateral views. It is important to evaluate both the AP and lateral views for a reverse rectosigmoid ratio, because it may not always be evident on both views. Although a reverse rectosigmoid ratio is highly suspicious for HD, that diagnosis was ruled out with rectal biopsy.

QUESTION 19.2

What would you do next?

A. Repeat contrast study
B. Anorectal manometry (AMAN)
C. Colonic manometry (CMAN)
D. Repeat rectal biopsy

Answer: Anorectal manometry should be performed to evaluate the functioning of this patient's internal and external sphincters (Answer B). Anorectal manometry testing done by gastroenterology showed an absent rectoanal inhibitory reflex (RAIR), which led to a diagnosis of internal sphincter achalasia. Internal sphincter achalasia is very typical in HD patients, but can also occur in other constipated patients without HD.

QUESTION 19.3

What does a diagnosis of internal sphincter achalasia mean?

Answer: Internal anal sphincter achalasia (IAS) is defined as a lack of the normal RAIR in patients who have a biopsy that shows ganglion cells. An absent RAIR is commonly seen in HD, but the presence of ganglion cells on full thickness rectal biopsy definitively rules out HD. Patients with an absent RAIR have internal anal sphincters that do not relax in response to stool descending into the rectum, which inhibits adequate stool evacuation.

With the AMAN findings of IAS, the sphincter problem could have been treated first with consideration to do CMAN testing in the future to evaluate for colonic dysmotility as the cause of his constipation if symptoms did not improve. However, colonic manometry had already been performed prior to presenting to our clinic, which showed somewhat disorganized high amplitude propagating contractions (HAPCs), and was interpreted as abnormal and suggestive of mild neuropathic dysmotility.

QUESTION 19.4

What should the next steps be?

A. Repeat rectal biopsy
B. Exam under anesthesia alone
C. Exam under anesthesia with Botulinum toxin
D. Exam under anesthesia with ileostomy

Answer: Based on this patient's severe, refractory constipation and failure to thrive, his previous response to Botulinum toxin, and the CMAN findings of dysmotility, we chose to proceed with an exam under anesthesia to rule out an anatomical cause of the obstructive symptoms and an ileostomy creation to bypass the obstructed/dysmotile colon and allow the patient to gain weight (Answer D). Although Botulinum toxin is commonly helpful in treating patients with IAS, this patient had previously received multiple Botulinum toxin injections to his anal canal without much improvement, so we omitted this from his treatment plan.

SIX MONTH FOLLOW-UP VISIT

The patient is growing well and gaining weight since having the ileostomy; however, his stool is still quite thick and he is struggling to pass stool through the ileostomy.

QUESTION 19.5

What can you do to facilitate adequate stooling through the ileostomy?

Answer: MiraLAX can help keep the stool soft and "flowing" to allow the patient's ileostomy to evacuate stool.

QUESTION 19.6

What additional testing might you consider given the patient's persistent hard stools via the ileostomy?

Answer: Due to the previous CMAN findings of disorganized HAPCs and possible neuropathic dysmotility, repeat CMAN as well as an assessment of the upper GI tract was performed. The CMAN findings now showed normal colonic motility. Antroduodenal manometry was also done to evaluate for dysmotility in the upper tract due to thick stools from ileostomy, which was also normal. At this time, the patient's severe obstructive symptoms were thought to be primarily due to his internal sphincter achalasia with the colonic dilation caused by his chronic constipation considered an important factor as well.

QUESTION 19.7

What is your next step to help treat this patient's obstructive symptoms?

- **A.** Botulinum toxin to the internal anal sphincter only
- **B.** Sigmoid resection + ileostomy closure
- **C.** Botulinum toxin + ileostomy closure
- **D.** Transanal rectosigmoid resection followed by Botulinum toxin, ileostomy closure, and antegrade flush option

Answer: We chose the following surgical plan:

- Transanal sigmoid pull through was done to remove the dilated rectum and sigmoid colon. A transanal rectal resection (as opposed to a sigmoid resection only) was performed given his Hirschsprung-like behavior to help improve motility and facilitate easier stool clearance.
- The patient recovered well following the initial surgery. After 4 months' time, he underwent ileostomy closure, Botulinum toxin injection of the internal sphincter to relax the internal sphincter achalasia, and Malone appendicostomy to allow for antegrade flushes. We chose to give the patient an antegrade flush option to allow for optimal daily stool clearance given his history of constipation with failure to thrive (Answer D).

As previously discussed, Botulinum toxin alone was not felt to be the best treatment for this patient given his poor response to previous injections, so Botulinum toxin alone with or without an ileostomy closure would not have worked for this patient. We also did not want to close the ileostomy at the same time as his resection because we wanted to monitor his recovery from the pull-through to ensure that he would be able to clear mucous and thrive first and to allow the coloanal anastomosis to heal.

ONE MONTH POSTOPERATIVE VISIT

The patient presented for his one month postoperative clinic visit. He was doing well with Malone flushes with 400 mL of saline and 20 mL of glycerin. He was tolerating the flushes well and was not having accidents. His X-ray from this visit is shown in Figure 19.3.

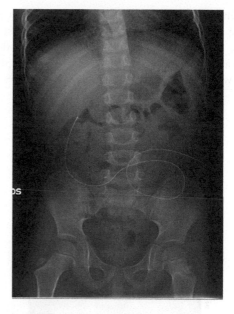

Figure 19.3 One month postoperative X-ray.

QUESTION 19.8

What is your assessment of the X-ray?

- **A.** Clean X-ray
- **B.** Impacted
- **C.** Stool in the rectum only
- **D.** Stool in the right colon and rectum

Answer: This patient's X-ray showed stool in the rectum and ascending colon (Answer D).

QUESTION 19.9

What would be your next step in this patient's care?

Answer: Our plan was to increase his flush strength to 450 mL of saline, 20 mL of glycerin, and 9 mL of Castile soap to empty the colon more effectively.

THREE MONTH POSTOPERATIVE VISIT

The patient presented for another follow-up visit three months postoperatively. His current regimen was Malone flushes with 450 mL of saline, 20 mL of glycerin, and 9 mL Castile soap. He was not having accidents and was tolerating the flushes well. He was having some difficulty getting stool out with flushes, and reporting straining during the flush as well as intermittent abdominal distention. His X-ray from this visit is seen in Figure 19.4, which was taken several hours after a flush.

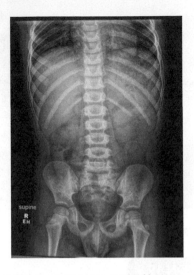

Figure 19.4 Three month postoperative X-ray.

QUESTION 19.10

What is your assessment of this X-ray? Why is the timing of the X-ray important when evaluating the efficiency of a flush?

Answer: The X-ray is clean with the exception of a small amount of stool in the right colon. This X-ray was taken several hours after a flush, so it is normal to see some stool buildup in the ascending colon.

QUESTION 19.11

What is your plan moving forward? What, if any, changes would you make to the flush? What other interventions might you consider?

Answer: Because this patient's X-ray was essentially clean several hours after a flush and he was doing well, we left the flush the same, 450 mL of saline, 20 mL of glycerin, and 9 mL of Castile. If this X-ray had been taken immediately following a flush, we may have considered increasing the strength of the flush to completely clean the colon.

We also have to consider this patient's worsening difficulty pushing out stool and need to remember his sphincter dysfunction. His last botulinum toxin injection was approximately 3 months prior to this encounter. It is likely that the effects of the botulinum toxin are wearing off at this point, as it typically lasts 3–4 months. Our plan moving forward was to schedule the patient for a repeat botulinum toxin injection.

DIFFICULTY EMPTYING AFTER REPEAT BOTULINUM TOXIN INJECTION

Approximately 1 week following a repeat Botulinum toxin injection to the anal sphincter, the patient presented with persistent difficulty emptying on his current flush regimen and reported increased accidents. The X-ray taken immediately following the patient's flush of 450 mL of saline, 20 mL of glycerin, and 9 mL of Castile soap is shown in Figure 19.5.

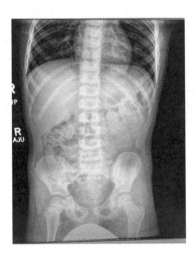

Figure 19.5 X-ray 1 week post-repeat botulinum toxin.

This patient's X-ray shows stool in the right colon and transverse colon despite just having completed a flush.

QUESTION 19.12

What is your plan moving forward?

A. Continue same regimen
B. Increase the current stimulants
C. Trial a different combination of stimulants
D. Decrease current stimulants

Answer: After seeing the updated X-ray, we reviewed the patient's repeat CMAN to see how he responded to the stimulants given. He had a very good response to bisacodyl during the CMAN. Therefore, we changed his flush to 450 mL of saline, 20 mL of glycerin, and 10 mg (30 mL) of bisacodyl (Answer C).

FOLLOW-UP VISIT FOLLOWING REGIMEN CHANGE

After switching to the new regimen, the patient was seen for follow-up. He was doing very well with flushes, reporting a good appetite, eating and growing well, tolerating the flush regimen, and not having accidents between flushes. His follow-up X-ray, taken 12 hours after his last flush is shown in Figure 19.6.

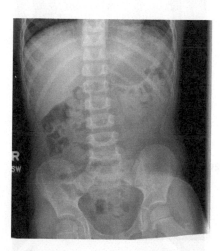

Figure 19.6 X-ray following regimen change to bisacodyl.

QUESTION 19.13

What is your assessment of the X-ray, and what is your plan moving forward?

Answer: The X-ray shows some stool in the right colon, which is expected 12 hours after a flush. The patient was doing well, therefore our plan moving forward was to keep him on his current regimen of 450 mL of saline, 20 mL of glycerin, and 10 mg (30 mL) of bisacodyl. He has continued to do well on this regimen, and his weight has increased from the 3rd percentile when we initially saw him to the 17th percentile.

KEY LEARNING POINTS

1. Contrast images, motility testing, physical exam, and biopsy results are all important components to evaluate a patient with refractory constipation.
2. Internal sphincter achalasia often requires regular Botulinum toxin injections (typically every 3 months or so) to promote relaxation of the sphincter and allow for adequate emptying.
3. Patients with chronic constipation (regardless of cause) are at risk for failure to thrive. A temporary ileostomy for a patient with severe, chronic constipation and failure to thrive (FTT) can help improve their appetite and allow for dramatic improvement in growth and development.
4. Patients with chronic constipation can have dilated segments of the colon, which slows down motility and causes worsening constipation. A resection of the dilated segment can help improve stool transit in these patients.
5. An antegrade option can help facilitate adequate stool clearance in patients who are prone to chronic constipation, and allows for more independence as the patient grows older compared to rectal enemas.
6. When determining a patient's regimen, the CMAN report can be especially helpful. If a patient has a strong response to a given stimulant during CMAN, it is helpful to start with that stimulant in their regimen first.
7. Assessment of colonic motility can be done by colonic manometry if available, but a nuclear medicine study is also very helpful as an alternative. Essentially, you need to know which of three situations a patient has: (1) normal motility; (2) segmental dysmotility (usually the sigmoid); or (3) diffuse dysmotility.

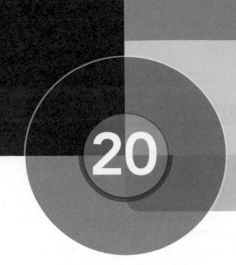

20

A patient with severe functional constipation, fecal impaction, and no soiling

JULIE ZIPFEL AND MARC A. LEVITT

CASE HISTORY

A 4-year-old boy with functional constipation and episodes of fecal impaction beginning at 2 months of age comes to clinic for evaluation. He has just started potty training, has one bowel movement per week, and his parents have noted some blood in the stool with pain on defecation. The parents have previously tried 1 capful (17 g) of polyethylene glycol 3350 daily with no change in his stooling pattern, and currently he is not on any bowel regimen.

QUESTION 20.1

What do you think of the medical treatment thus far?

Answer: The child's bowel care has not been sufficiently addressed. He would benefit from a bowel management program that leads to a daily bowel movement. His rectum should be examined for any anatomic abnormalities. Botulinum toxin injection could be a consideration and may be of benefit if there is a withholding or sphincter dysfunction concern. The child is having just one bowel movement per week with blood in the stool. The use of MiraLAX, an osmotic laxative, works by bringing water into the bowel; however, if the child is already impacted, stool will eventually harden and worsen the stool accumulation.

As part of his evaluation, a contrast enema is performed (see Figures 20.1 and 20.2).

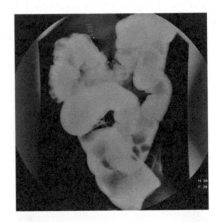

Figure 20.1 Contrast enema.

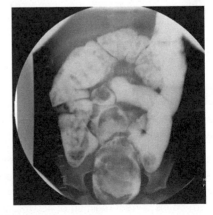

Figure 20.2 Contrast enema.

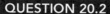

QUESTION 20.2

What does the contrast enema show?

Answer: The contrast enema shows a mild generalized distention of the rectosigmoid and sigmoid redundancy most compatible with functional constipation. There is generalized fecal retention. There is a normal colonic rotation, and no focal stricture.

QUESTION 20.3

What would happen over time if the constipation were to continue to not be adequately managed?

Answer: Over time, the rectum becomes stretched, much like a balloon loses its tensile strength, in a vicious cycle—more constipation leads to more distention, which leads to more constipation. Several situations can occur—rectal prolapse (either internal intussusception, external prolapse or internal prolapse); additionally, the rectum and sigmoid become progressively more dilated, and the nerves within the rectal complex could become hypertrophied causing loss of sensation, urge, and muscle tone within the sphincter and they become weakened and this can lead to leakage of stool.

After insuring that the colon was clean, the child was begun on a bowel regimen of 15 mg of senna daily. Senna will help to keep water within the intestine, softening stool and stimulating bowel movement. An abdominal X-ray was planned in 1 week to assess the stool load.

Changes in routine, poor diet, hydration status, and increased stress levels are perpetuating factors that induce varying outcomes in children with functional constipation. Education for parents addressing compliance, medication dosing, activity, and diet may aid in enhancing outcomes.

STOOL SOFTENER VS. LAXATIVE

Both stool softeners and laxatives can aid in the relief of constipation. Knowledge regarding the classification, effectiveness, function, and side effects of bowel management preparations are beneficial for optimal bowel emptying (Table 20.1).

LAXATIVES

Table 20.1 Laxatives and stool softeners

Laxatives classification	Effectiveness	Function	Side effects
Bulk-forming	For larger stool—makes bowel contract	Contains fiber which uses the water within the intestines to bulk up the stool	Bloating and gas
Stimulant	Pushes stool out	Increased peristalsis	Stomach discomfort, cramps, faintness
Osmotic-PEG (polyethylene glycol)	Soften stools, increases bowel movements	Draws water into the bowel	Nausea, bloating, cramping, gas
Lubricant	Stools retain fluid and pass more easily	Coats stool with an oily/greasy residue	Inhibits absorption of vitamins and nutrients

Note: One should never give laxatives and enemas at the same time, except if an enema is needed to clear an impaction.

At 1 week, the child is having one bowel movement per day, but it is reported to be watery. An X-ray is performed (Figure 20.3).

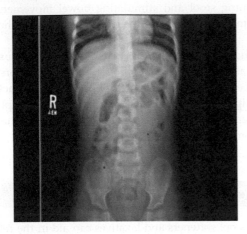

Figure 20.3 Abdominal X-ray.

QUESTION 20.4

How would you interpret the abdominal X-ray?

Answer: The overall stool volume is mild. The bowel gas pattern is normal.

QUESTION 20.5

Would you make any adjustments to the bowel regimen at this time?

Answer: For the next week, add water-soluble fiber to the child's regimen. An increase in water-soluble fiber will absorb water within the colon and help to bulk up the stool, as the stimulant laxative continues to work, but now on more bulked-up stool.

At 2 weeks, the patient returns for an office visit. His current regimen is 15 mg senna daily, and 3 g of water-soluble fiber twice a day. He is having a bowel movement every other day, which has become formed again, not hard. He currently has no abdominal pain or vomiting; however, the parents are both witnessing signs of withholding and straining. At this time anorectal manometry (AMAN) would be beneficial to assess the pressures of the anal sphincter muscles, rectal sensation, and nerve reflex, all of which are necessary for elimination. Additionally, exam under anesthesia and possible botulinum toxin, based on the AMAN results, may be indicated.

QUESTION 20.6

What advice can you give to the parents regarding withholding?

Answer: Withholding can be a sign of stress due to fear and/or pain from passing large bowel movements. Information for parents would include monitoring the child's diet (certain foods can make stools hard, see Table 20.2) and use positive reinforcement to alleviate additional stressors.

CONSTIPATING FOODS

Table 20.2 Diet that leads to constipation

Milk	All milk products allowed, but limit to 500 mL total per day
Vegetables	Vegetable juice without pulp, well cooked vegetables, green beans, spinach, pumpkin, eggplant, potatoes without skin, asparagus, beets, carrots
Fruits	Applesauce, apples (without skin), banana, melon
Starch, grains	Bread, crackers, cereals made from refined flours, pasta or noodles made from white flour, white rice, pretzels, white potatoes (without skin), dry cereal
Meat, seafood, legumes	Baked/broiled/grilled meats, poultry or fish, lean deli meats, eggs
Fats, oils	Butter, margarine, oils, fried foods
Sweets	Sugar-free gelatin, popsicles, jelly, or syrup, rice-milk ice cream
Beverages	Water, sugar-free Gatorade, sugar-free Crystal Light, sugar-free Kool-Aid, Pedialyte

The child returns to your office at one month follow-up. His current regimen is 15 mg of senna daily, and 3 g of fiber twice a day. He had been having bowel movements every other day but on this day he has not had a stool in 3 days. He has had an AMAN performed in the interval which reveals anal sphincter achalasia, a condition where the internal sphincter cannot relax. The child was scheduled for anal botulinum toxin injection and will follow-up in 4 months. This injection of the anal sphincter will allow the sphincter to relax thereby allowing defecation and reducing stool accumulation within the colon. He will eventually learn how to relax his sphincters at the appropriate time. He will continue on 15 mg of senna daily, and 3 g of fiber twice a day.

LAXATIVE FOODS

Please refer to Table 20.3.

Table 20.3 Foods that produce a laxative effect

Milk	High-fat dairy products, such as whole milk, yogurt, or cottage cheese
Vegetables	All vegetables (raw vegetables are best)
Fruits	All fruits, fruit juice with pulp, canned pineapple, prunes, dried fruit, jam, marmalade, dried fruits
Starch, grains	Wholegrain or seeded breads, wholegrain pasta and cereal, brown rice, oatmeal, and bran cereal
Meat, seafood, legumes	Beans, fried or greasy meats, salami, cold cuts, hot dogs, meat substitutes
Fats, oils	Butter, margarine, oils, fried foods
Sweets	Chocolate (dark chocolate is the best)
Beverages	Soda, juices, high-sugar drinks, Kool-Aid®, powdered drinks
Seasonings	Oregano, rosemary, marjoram, basil, fennel, paprika, thyme

KEY LEARNING POINTS

1. Provide reassurance along with positive reinforcement to a child who is showing signs of withholding. Take steps to keep stool soft. Most children will hold stool because they have had a prior large bowel movement that was painful.
2. Education should be done with the family regarding the patient's diet. It would be beneficial for the family to keep a food journal (diary) to see which foods may be causing the trigger for the constipation. Encouraging specific foods vs. restriction of foods is often met with more acceptance.

SUGGESTED READINGS

Ahmadi, J., Azary, S., Ashjaei, B., Paragomi, P., & Khalifeh-Soltani, A. 2013. Intrasphincteric botulinum toxin injection in treatment of chronic idiopathic constipation in children. *Iranian Journal of Pediatrics*, 23(5), 574–578.

Gonzalez-Martinez, M. A., Ortiz-Olvera, N. X., & Mendez-Navarro, J. 2013. Novel pharmacological therapies for management of chronic constipation. *Journal of Clinical Gastroenterology*, 48(1), 21–28.

Levy, E. I., Lemmens, R., Vandenplas, Y., & Devreker, T. 2017. Functional constipation in children: Challenges and solutions. *Pediatric Health, Medicine and Therapeutics*, 8, 19–27.

Vilanova-Sanchez, A., Gasior, A. C., Toocheck, N. et al. 2018. Are senna based laxatives safe when used as long term treatment for constipation in children? *Journal of Pediatric Surgery*, 53(4), 722–727.

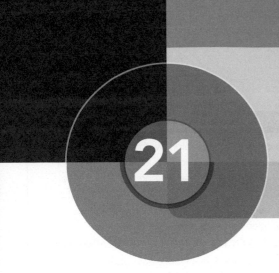

A patient with severe functional constipation, fecal impaction, and soiling

21

JULIE ZIPFEL AND MARC A. LEVITT

CASE HISTORY

A 10-year-old male with a history of functional constipation and fecal soiling since birth comes to your clinic. He soils daily. His past medical history is significant for attention deficit hyperactivity disorder, oppositional defiant disorder, and sexual molestation with resultant anal defensiveness. He has had chronic constipation since the age of 1. At age 9, he had anal dilation and anal botulinum toxin at another institution for withholding behavior with no improvement in his symptoms. He has tried polyethylene glycol 3350 and senna, but this resulted in significant cramping, decreased appetite, and multiple daily accidents. He has been hospitalized twice in the last 3 months for impactions requiring a GoLYTELY cleanout.

QUESTION 21.1

What could be the cause of the cramping, decreased appetite, and daily accidents after using MiraLAX and senna?

Answer: High dose laxative use can cause significant side effects (e.g., nausea, vomiting, bloating, and abdominal pain), particularly if the colon is full when these medication are given.

QUESTION 21.2

A previous magnetic resonance imaging (MRI) had been performed. What would be the rationale for this exam?

Answer: In pediatric patients with chronic constipation, an MRI can reveal abnormalities in the lumbar spine. While a neurologic examination may prove normal, a tethered cord, spina bifida occulta, or fatty filum (>2 mm at L5-S1) may be present, and could be the cause of neurogenic bowel. In patients with severe constipation that is refractory to medical management, this study should be considered.

QUESTION 21.3

How would you interpret these findings?

Answer: The spinal MRI shows a disc bulge at L5-S1, and no tethered cord or other spinal anomalies. The patient is currently not complaining of back pain, numbness or tingling, with or without radiation to his lower extremities. The findings were considered an incidental finding. Should future symptoms occur, further follow-up would be warranted (Figures 21.1 and 21.2).

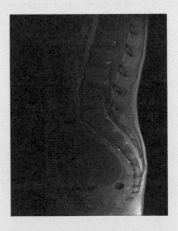

Figure 21.1 Lateral spinal MRI.

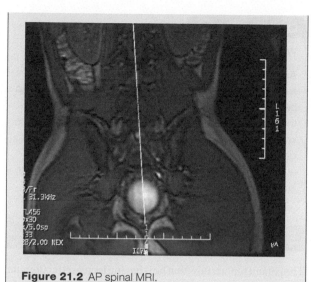

Figure 21.2 AP spinal MRI.

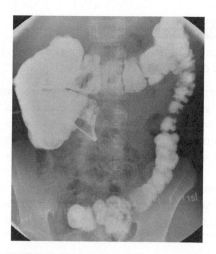

Figure 21.3 Contrast enema.

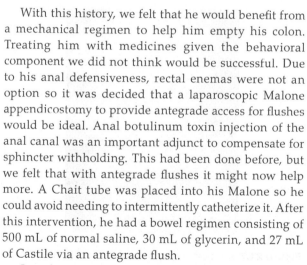

Figure 21.4 Contrast enema.

With this history, we felt that he would benefit from a mechanical regimen to help him empty his colon. Treating him with medicines given the behavioral component we did not think would be successful. Due to his anal defensiveness, rectal enemas were not an option so it was decided that a laparoscopic Malone appendicostomy to provide antegrade access for flushes would be ideal. Anal botulinum toxin injection of the anal canal was an important adjunct to compensate for sphincter withholding. This had been done before, but we felt that with antegrade flushes it might now help more. A Chait tube was placed into his Malone so he could avoid needing to intermittently catheterize it. After this intervention, he had a bowel regimen consisting of 500 mL of normal saline, 30 mL of glycerin, and 27 mL of Castile via an antegrade flush.

Over the next several months, he was having hard stools with very little output most days. A bowel management program was recommended to fine-tune the flush regimen to help eliminate the daily accidents.

The patient comes for a bowel management program and a contrast enema is ordered prior to this visit to assess the antegrade flush (Figures 21.3 through 21.5).

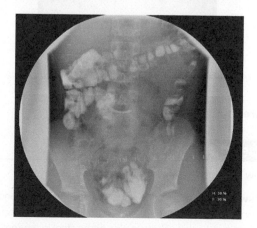

Figure 21.5 Post-evacuation film.

QUESTION 21.4

How do you interpret the findings on the contrast enema done via the Malone?

Answer: The contrast enema shows minimal stool in the cecum and rectum. A tube in his Malone projects over the right hemiabdomen. A normal caliber colon is noted from the cecum to the rectosigmoid with the cecum slightly larger in caliber than the rest of the colon. There is no stricture or dilation. A normal rectosigmoid is observed with peristalsis. There is no reflux into the terminal ileum. The post-evacuation image reveals no bowel distention, and the majority of the contrast has been expelled.

BOWEL MANAGEMENT DAY 1

The patient arrives to the clinic for day 1 of the bowel management program to fine-tune his regimen and improve emptying. He has done his morning antegrade flush using saline 500 mL, glycerin 30 mL, and Castile 27 mL (Figure 21.6).

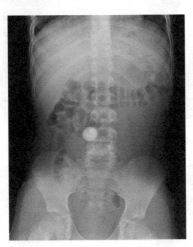

Figure 21.6 Abdominal X-ray.

QUESTION 21.5

How would you interpret his morning X-ray?

Answer: The abdominal X-ray shows stool in the ascending colon, and an otherwise normal transverse, descending, and sigmoid colon. There is also some stool in the rectum, and there is a normal bowel gas pattern.

QUESTION 21.6

Would you make any regimen changes at this time?

Answer: With stool persisting in the rectum even after the flush this morning a regimen change is done in an effort to better clean the colon. Bisacodyl 30 mL, wait 5–10 minutes, then administer 400 mL of saline will be tried. Bisacodyl use will induce contractions within the bowel; it is considered to be a stronger stimulant laxative than glycerin. The delay in administering the flush will allow the bisacodyl to work on its own before dilution by the 400 mL normal saline flush.

BOWEL MANAGEMENT DAY 2

The patient reports now that he is having increased abdominal pain after 10 minutes of instilling his bisacodyl flush, and he had four accidents during the night (Figure 21.7).

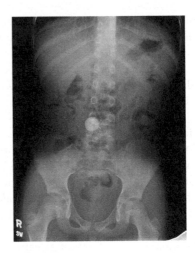

Figure 21.7 Abdominal X-ray.

QUESTION 21.7

How would you interpret his day 2 morning X-ray?

Answer: A Mic-key button is present over the L4-L5 disc space which was placed instead of the Chait. We felt this tube was preferable as it has a balloon device that helps to prevent leakage. There are no dilated loops or signs of obstruction. There is persistence of stool in the right colon. There is scattered stool extending from the splenic flexure to the pelvis. There is no impaction or dilation.

QUESTION 21.8

Would you do a regimen change at this time?

Answer: With the persistence of stool within the colon a regimen change is warranted to achieve a cleaner colon. The patient is told to lie on his right side and instill 45 mL of bisacodyl 20 minutes prior to his 400 mL tap water flush. A switch to tap water is being tried to see if it will make any difference in the patient's cramping symptoms, which could be due to the saline. Each child is unique, therefore varying approaches must be tried with each child until a successful bowel regimen is identified. When using tap water, it is important to watch for signs of dehydration and electrolyte imbalance, specifically hyponatremia, which is mostly relevant in young children (under age 3). Additionally, having the patient lie on his right side during the 20-minute wait time may help to dissolve the stool therein.

BOWEL MANAGEMENT DAY 5

It is mid-week of the bowel management program. The patient reports having increased abdominal pain and multiple accidents during the night (Figure 21.8).

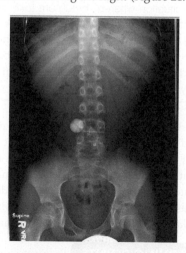

Figure 21.8 Abdominal X-ray.

QUESTION 21.9

How would you interpret this abdominal X-ray?

Answer: There is mild to moderate volume of stool noted throughout the colon. There is a normal distribution of bowel gas and no dilated loops.

QUESTION 21.10

What suggestions based on his report and this X-ray would you make on managing his flushes to decrease nighttime stooling?

Answer: By adjusting his first flush time to earlier in the afternoon he will have more time to empty prior to bedtime and this should decrease his bedtime accidents.

QUESTION 21.11

Would you adjust his regimen at this time?

Answer: More strength to his regimen is needed to try to get him cleaned out. Bisacodyl 45 mL mixed directly with 400 mL of normal saline will be done twice today, with the goal of getting him completely emptied. A regimen change was planned for tomorrow using 400 ml of tap water and increasing bisacodyl to 60 ml once daily. Once the colon is clean again, adjustments can be made based on his daily abdominal X-ray and the hope of keeping him clean for 24 hours between enemas.

BOWEL MANAGEMENT DAY 6 (FIGURE 21.9)

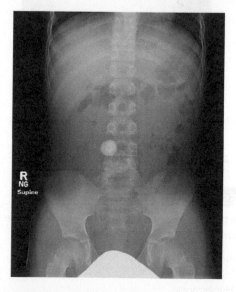

Figure 21.9 Abdominal X-ray.

QUESTION 21.12

The patient is clean with minimal cramping. How would you interpret today's X-ray compared to the prior day's X-ray?

A. Decreased stool
B. Unchanged
C. Increased stool

Answer: The X-ray shows minimal stool in the ascending colon with no significant stool throughout the transverse, descending, sigmoid colon, or within the rectum. The X-ray has decreased stool burden from the prior day's abdominal X-ray (Answer A). No regimen change should be made at this time. Continue with 400 mL of tap water plus 60 mL of bisacodyl once daily.

BOWEL MANAGEMENT DAY 7 (FIGURE 21.10)

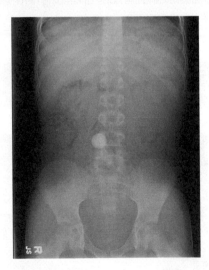

Figure 21.10 Abdominal X-ray.

QUESTION 21.13

From the X-rays presented, how would you assess the patient's motility?

A. Normal
B. Hypomotile
C. Hypermotile

Answer: The patient's colon has accumulated stool again. The patient has a slow-moving colon (hypomotile) (Answer B). Hypomotility results in decreased contractility within the colon and results in chronic constipation.

A regimen change is done today, as well as some additional testing. We started the patient on 400 mL of normal saline and increased the bisacodyl to 90 mL daily.

QUESTION 21.14

What testing should be done to better assess motility given the difficulty you are having emptying his colon?

A. Anorectal manometry (AMAN)
B. Colonic manometry catheter placement via cecostomy (CMAN)
C. Both A and B

Answer: The patient would benefit from both an AMAN and a CMAN (Answer C). AMAN will measure the contractility in the anus and rectum to determine the presence or absence of the rectosphincteric reflex. This reflex is responsible for relaxation of the internal anal sphincter when the rectum distends allowing evacuation of stool. If abnormal, it may indicate a situation whereby botulinum toxin injection of the sphincter can improve colonic emptying. A CMAN will determine how well the muscles in the large intestine are contracting; this contraction allows stool to be expelled and can determine whether a specific segment of the colon is dysmotile.

Results of the AMAN reveal a completely normal anal sphincter. The CMAN suggests colonic inertia diffusely, throughout the entire colon. This is a rare dysmotility disorder causing slow transit of the colon and requiring surgical intervention. Options would include diverting ileostomy as an initial step and possibly total abdominal colectomy later, with a right colon to rectum anastomosis.

KEY LEARNING POINTS

1. There are no known pathophysiological causes of functional constipation/chronic idiopathic constipation. Factors that potentiate constipation include: major life events and behavioral disorders. Additionally, children's exposure to abuse or maltreatment may affect the clinician's options for management of their constipation.

2. Remember that each patient is unique. The approach during a bowel management program is to fine-tune a regimen that the patient and family will be most amenable to during the visit and then when back at home. Adjustments in the flush—normal saline or water, glycerin, soap or bisacodyl, etc.—all can be used to fine-tune the flush. Abdominal X-rays are performed throughout the week to verify if the regimen has been effective. If ineffective, changes in the plan, sometimes on a daily basis, will be done until the colon is successfully emptied and the patient stops having accidents.

3. The goal of the bowel management week is to get the patient clean; however, despite our bowel management protocol there are times when it does not work, and further follow-up via testing (anorectal manometry, colonic manometry) will need to be done to rule out other findings which would require more aggressive treatments.

4. AMAN looks for the presence or absence of an anal inhibitory response. If absent, this would be suggestive of Hirschsprung disease. Rectal biopsy in such a case should be performed to confirm the presence or absence of ganglion cells. If ganglion cells are found to be present this would be indicative of internal sphincter achalasia, a condition in which the internal anal sphincter is unable to relax. This condition has been shown to be successfully treated with botulinum toxin injections into the rectal sphincter, allowing relaxation of the muscle complex.

5. CMAN is a study used to determine the presence and strength of contractions via the muscles within the colon. The results of the CMAN are useful to guide treatment options such as antegrade flush options and whether a colon resection is warranted.

SUGGESTED READINGS

Ahmadi, J., Azary, S., Ashjaei, B., Paragomi, P., & Khalifeh-Soltani, A. 2013. Intrasphincteric botulinum toxin injection in treatment of chronic idiopathic constipation in children. *Iranian Journal of Pediatrics*, 23(5), 574–578.

Dinning, P. G., Benninga, M. A., Southwell, B. R., & Scott, S. M. 2010. Paediatric and adult colonic manometry: A tool to help unravel the pathophysiology of constipation. *World Journal of Gastroenterology*, 16(41), 5162–5172.

Koppen, I. J. N., Lammers, L. A., Benninga, M. A., & Tabbers, M. M. 2015. Management of functional constipation in children: Therapy in practice. *Paediatric Drugs*, 17, 349–360.

McCoy, J. A. & Beck, D. E. 2012. Surgical management of colonic inertia. *Clinics in Colon and Rectal Surgery*, 25(1), 20–23.

Rajindrajith, S., Devanarayana, N. M., & Benninga, M. A. 2017. Association between child maltreatment and constipation: A school-based survey using rome III criteria, *Journal of Pediatric Gastroenterology & Nutrition*. 58(4), 486–490, April 2014.

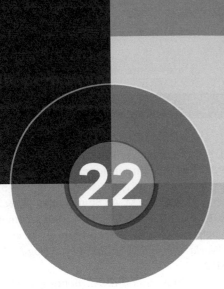

A patient with a successful rectal enema regimen but who now is unable to tolerate rectal administration

ANDREA WAGNER

CASE HISTORY

A 15-year-old male with functional constipation and fecal incontinence since the age of 4 presents to your clinic. He typically has one large and hard bowel movement every 4–5 days and a small volume soiling daily. He has tried senna and lactulose regimens without success. He voids normally, has no urinary incontinence during the day or night, and has no history of urinary tract infections. He has a history of autism and is currently in the custody of a family friend. He has no past surgical history.

Initial evaluation of this child revealed a normal physical exam. A contrast enema via rectum (Figure 22.1) is shown below.

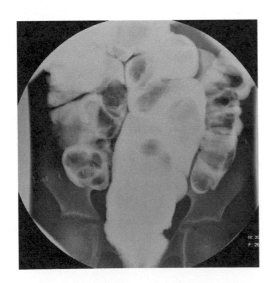

Figure 22.1 Contrast enema.

QUESTION 22.1

How would you describe and interpret the findings on the contrast enema?

Answer: Key findings include a dilated vertically oriented rectum and sigmoid colon extending to the hepatic flexure. There is redundancy of the sigmoid colon as well. There is subtle spiculation of the rectum suggesting smooth muscle work hypertrophy of the rectum (jejunalization). These findings, coupled with his history and exam, suggest that this child has longstanding constipation with pseudo-incontinence.

QUESTION 22.2

What type of bowel management regimen would best address this child's soiling?

Answer: Two main treatment modalities, rectal enemas and oral laxatives were discussed with the child and his care provider. The family and patient felt he had already tried several oral treatment regimens without success. The decision was made to start him on a rectal enema regimen with the understanding that this treatment modality would provide the faster, more reliable and predictable route to end his soiling.

During bowel management week, he was started on a bowel regimen of daily rectal enema with 500 mL of saline and 30 mL of glycerin.

On day 1 of bowel management week, the patient reports good stool output following the enema, but with stool leakage overnight.

QUESTION 22.3

What does his X-ray reveal (Figure 22.2)?

Answer: There is marked residual contrast on his day 1 X-ray following administration of the enema with 500 mL of saline and 30 mL of glycerin.

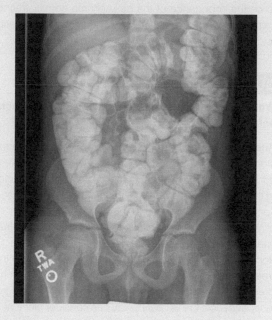

Figure 22.2 Abdominal X-ray.

QUESTION 22.4

What is your plan for day 2 of bowel management week given this history and X-ray?

Answer: Increase the volume of the rectal enema to 600 mL of saline and 30 mL of glycerin.
On day 2 of bowel management week, the patient reports good stool output following the enema, but slightly less volume than on day 1. He again has stool leakage overnight.

QUESTION 22.5

What does his X-ray reveal (Figure 22.3)?

Answer: There is persistent residual contrast on the X-ray.

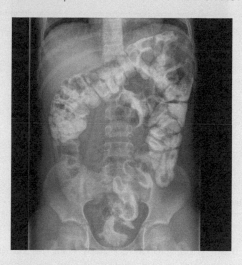

Figure 22.3 Abdominal X-ray.

QUESTION 22.6

What is your plan for day 3 of bowel management week given this history and X-ray?

Answer: Increase the amount of stimulant to increase the overall strength of the enema regimen. New regimen:
600 mL of saline, 30 mL of glycerin, and 9 mL of Castile soap.
On days 4–7 of bowel management week, the patient reports excellent stool output following the enema. He denies nausea, vomiting or abdominal pain. He has had no soiling in his pull ups overnight.

QUESTION 22.7

What does this X-ray from day 7 of bowel management show (Figure 22.4)?

Answer: This X-ray reveals excellent stool clearance from the rectosigmoid colon. Therefore, the enema of 600 mL of saline, 30 mL of glycerin, and 9 mL of Castile soap remained his regimen at the completion of his bowel management week. You ask the patient to return in 1 month.

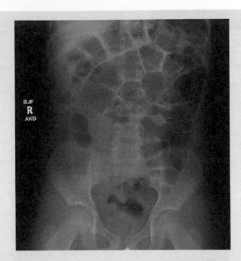

Figure 22.4 Abdominal X-ray.

At the 1 month follow-up clinic visit, the patient and the care provider, a maternal great aunt, describe waxing dedication to the once daily enema regimen. The patient denies fecal soiling.

QUESTION 22.8

What does his X-ray reveal (Figure 22.5)?

Answer: The X-ray reveals residual stool following the enema in the rectosigmoid colon.

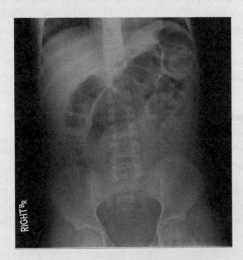

Figure 22.5 Abdominal X-ray.

QUESTION 22.9

Would you make any changes in the short-term to his regimen given the history and X-ray findings?

Answer: Because he is not adhering to the daily prescription stool may be accumulating over time. You must reinforce the importance of the daily enema administration. Increase strength to 600 mL of saline, 30 mL of glycerin, and 18 mL of Castile soap. Follow-up in 2 weeks.

QUESTION 22.10

What can you do regarding noncompliance with rectal enemas in this patient?

Answer: Talk with the patient and caregiver to best understand the reason for noncompliance. This child is able to adhere to a 30–45-minute sit time following administration of the enema. He tolerates the enema well without nausea, vomiting, or abdominal pain. He has good stool clearance clinically and radiographically. The treatment plan has eradicated his chronic soiling. Acknowledge that the rectal administration may be the most burdensome aspect of this treatment plan. This is particularly common in older children or adolescents who are appropriately trying to gain independence. In this patient, you can consider placement of a Malone appendicostomy for antegrade enema administration. The Malone appendicostomy allows the child to administer the same effective enema, and maintain privacy during flushes and independence with self-care.

This patient underwent Malone appendicostomy and is doing well with daily Malone flushes.

QUESTION 22.11

For such a patient, at what point might you consider testing with anorectal and colonic manometry?

Answer: The patient plans to do another bowel management week in the future, after 6 months of successful antegrade flushing, this time with an oral laxative regimen. Had the patient not been successful with oral laxatives or with enemas, you should consider referral for colonic and anorectal manometry testing. It is possible that he has colonic dysmotility and might benefit from a resection of dysmotile sigmoid colon. He may also have pelvic floor dysfunction and benefit from anal botulinum toxin injection or biofeedback to better coordinate his sphincter muscles.

KEY LEARNING POINTS

1. Allow older children to be active participants in their care plan. Help them understand the different treatment options, long-term plans, and reasoning behind medical decisions.

2. Rectal enemas do not have to be prescribed long term, but in some cases can be used as a trial prior to creation of Malone appendicostomy for antegrade enema administration or as a bridge until the patient is able to try or retry an oral laxative regimen.

3. After several months of successful rectal or antegrade enemas in a patient with functional constipation, you should repeat a bowel management week with laxatives if the patient and family is motivated to do so, and there are no behavioral limitations.

   a. The child may require a smaller laxative dose or be more successful with laxatives after compliance for a time with rectal enemas or antegrade enemas.

   b. If the patient does not experience success with reattempted laxatives, then such a patient should undergo further evaluation with anorectal and colonic manometry testing.

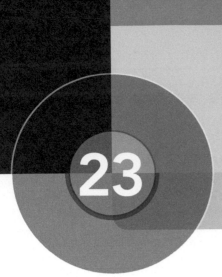
A patient with severe functional constipation who has failed laxative treatment and both rectal and antegrade enemas

JULIE GERBERICK

CASE HISTORY

An 8-year-old female is referred to your clinic for evaluation of her chronic constipation. She has a history of lifelong stooling problems. She currently has one bowel movement each day and complains of hard stool, abdominal pain, and straining. She has required inpatient hospitalizations twice this past year for a bowel cleanout. She takes the oral osmotic laxative polyethylene glycol 3350 (MiraLAX®) 17 g daily, the oral stimulant laxative senna 65 mg daily and a small volume over-the-counter saline rectal enema as needed. Despite these, she has fecal soiling three to four times a week. She urinates five to six times a day with complete control, but has urinary frequency, urgency, and urinary tract infections three to four times a year. She has been hospitalized once in the past year for pyelonephritis.

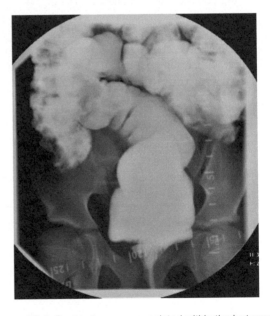

Figure 23.1 Contrast enema completed within the last year.

QUESTION 23.1

What is polyethylene glycol 3350 (MiraLAX®)? What is senna? How do their actions differ?

Answer: Polyethylene glycol 3350 is an oral osmotic laxative that makes stool soft, but does not help it come out. Senna is an oral stimulant laxative that promotes stooling, by inducing peristalsis. The starting senna dose is 1–2 mg/kg with a maximum dose based on the patient's tolerance and symptoms.

The child had a contrast enema in the past year, which is shown in Figure 23.1.

QUESTION 23.2

What are the findings on this contrast enema?

Answer: The contrast enema shows mild redundancy and dilation of the rectosigmoid.

QUESTION 23.3

What is your plan for this patient?

Answer: The child will benefit from a devoted bowel management program.

The X-ray in Figure 23.2 was obtained at the beginning of bowel management week.

What does this X-ray show with regard to stool volume?

Answer: The X-ray shows stool in the left colon and some stool in the right colon.

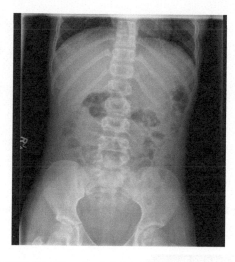

Figure 23.2 X-ray from the first day of bowel management week.

What would you do next?

Answer: It was decided to start this child on a once daily dose of the oral stimulant laxative senna 75 mg and water-soluble fiber 2 g daily. This senna dose was increased from her previous dose of 65 mg as she was having stool accidents four times each week and had the X-ray findings which we concluded meant she was not emptying her colon adequately (Figure 23.2). The water-soluble fiber was added to bulk the stool in the colon to improve the sensation of stool and decrease the number of stools each day. The laxative regimen was initiated rather than a rectal enema regimen as the family expressed significant concern with the administration of rectal medications or enemas.

The child had a renal ultrasound during bowel management week which was normal.

What recommendations should be made from a urologic point of view?

A. Importance of daily bowel movements to minimize retention of stool
B. Importance of daily cleansing of the perineum and introitus with soap and water to kill off the uropathogenic bacteria that may colonize in that area
C. Importance of voiding every 2–3 hours while awake
D. Importance of anticholinergics for overactive bladder
E. Importance of all the above

Answer: Recommendations would include the importance all of the above (Answer E) to decrease urinary retention, which may contribute to her urinary symptoms and urinary tract infections.

The child had varying results during bowel management week and had X-rays that showed either an increase in stool in the colon or a clean colon while on senna which was increased to 100 mg and then decreased back to 75 mg once daily over the course of the week with 2 g of water-soluble fiber added twice daily. The child complained of abdominal cramping and nausea throughout the week. She also had days with accidents and days with no accidents. Figure 23.3 shows her X-ray at the end of bowel management week.

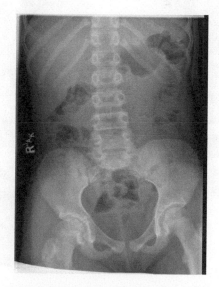

Figure 23.3 X-ray from the last day of bowel management week.

QUESTION 23.7

What does this X-ray show with regard to stool volume?

A. Stool in the right and left colon, but a clean rectum
B. No stool in the colon
C. Hard to tell with this image
D. Stool in the transverse colon but a clean rectosigmoid

Answer: The X-ray shows stool in the right and left colon, but a clean rectum (Answer A).

QUESTION 23.8

What would you do next?

Answer: It was determined to have the child complete the bowel management program week on the regimen of 75 mg of senna daily and 2 g of fiber twice daily to give her body time to adjust to a consistent regimen. The child was encouraged to sit on the toilet when she had the abdominal cramping to attempt to pass stool.

Over the course of the next several months, the child experienced decreased stool output and presented to the emergency department three times with abdominal pain, soiling, bloating, and impaction. Figures 23.4 and 23.5 show her X-ray images from one of these visits.

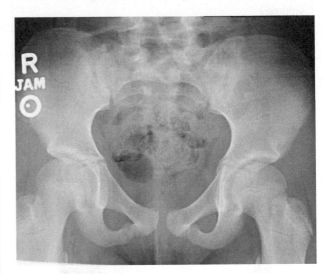

Figure 23.5 X-ray from emergency department visit, view of the pelvis.

QUESTION 23.9

What do the X-rays show? What would you do?

Answer: The X-ray shows moderate stool in her colon and a heavily impacted rectum. She was admitted to the hospital for a bowel cleanout and was discharged home after three days on 125 mg of senna, 68 g of the oral osmotic laxative polyethylene glycol 3350 once daily and 2 g of water-soluble fiber twice daily.

The child presents for follow-up and the family reports she is stooling one to two times per day. The stool is hard and she continues to have nausea, abdominal cramping, and daily stool accidents with leakage.

The X-ray image in Figure 23.6 was obtained.

Figure 23.4 X-ray from emergency department visit.

QUESTION 23.10

What does the X-ray show?

Answer: The X-ray shows a clean colon.

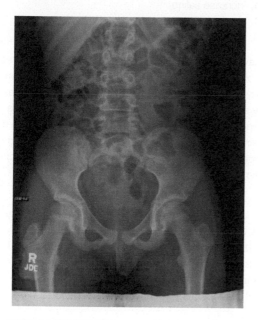

Figure 23.6 X-ray from follow-up clinic visit.

QUESTION 23.11

What changes would you make with the child's bowel regimen after reviewing this X-ray?

A. Increase the senna dose and polyethylene glycol 3350 dose
B. Decrease the senna dose and polyethylene glycol 3350 dose
C. Make no changes
D. Decrease the senna dose but increase the polyethylene glycol 3350 dose

Answer: The patient has a clean colon with abdominal cramping and stool accidents. You can conclude from this that she is being overstimulated and the decision was made to decrease the senna dose to 112.5 mg once daily and polyethylene glycol 3350 dose to 17 g daily (Answer B).

QUESTION 23.12

What is your next step?

Answer: Owing to the patient's ongoing clinical course with constipation requiring hospitalization, persistent accidents, abdominal pain, and several failed attempts at medical management, it was decided to obtain anorectal manometry and colonic manometry testing to evaluate for any sphincter or motility concerns, which may explain her failure of medical management.

Results of the patient's motility testing:

- *Anorectal manometry*: Intact rectoanal inhibitory reflex (RAIR), normal resting pressure, normal squeeze pressure, abnormal push test consistent with external anal sphincter dyssynergia
- *Colonic manometry*: Normal with multiple and strong propagating contractions post-stimulant throughout the colon

QUESTION 23.13

With the child's ongoing challenges with stimulant laxatives and the findings from the motility testing it was decided she would benefit from which of the following:

A. Anal botulinum toxin
B. Biofeedback therapy
C. Rectal enema option
D. Psychological support
E. All of the above

Answer: In collaboration with the gastroenterology/motility team it was decided that all of the above would be most appropriate for this child (Answer E). The child will first attend a second bowel management week to try rectal enemas, to see if she improves the symptoms of abdominal and rectal pain, and this could decrease the soiling.

The child started a second bowel management program week with rectal enemas of 500 mL of saline and 30 mL of glycerin. Oral laxatives were stopped. Her X-ray to begin the week showed stool throughout the colon with rectal stool distension (Figure 23.7).

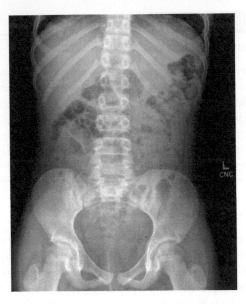

Figure 23.7 X-ray from the first day of the second bowel management week.

Mid-bowel management week on a rectal enema regimen of 500 mL of saline, 30 mL of glycerin, and 9 mL of Castile soap, the child had no fecal soiling, no abdominal distension or pain, and the results can be seen in the X-ray image in Figure 23.8.

QUESTION 23.14

What would the X-ray findings suggest should be the following regimen recommendations:

   A. Increase glycerin
   B. Increase saline
   C. Increase Castile soap
   D. Leave the regimen the same

Answer: Based on the X-ray with colonic and rectal stool burden, increasing the Castile soap is the correct answer (Answer C). We would not recommend increasing the saline volume or glycerin at this time. Increasing the saline volume would dilute the additives/irritants and may decrease the effectiveness of the flush. Increasing the glycerin may cause an increase in side effects such as cramping or nausea.

The child went home from the second bowel management week on a regimen of 500 mL of saline, 30 mL of glycerin, and 18 mL of Castile soap. She denied abdominal pain, nausea, or vomiting, and had no soiling. The child's X-ray demonstrated only a mild colonic stool burden at the end of bowel management as shown in Figure 23.9.

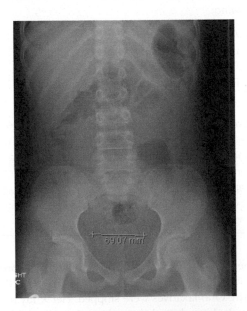

Figure 23.8 X-ray from the middle of the second bowel management week.

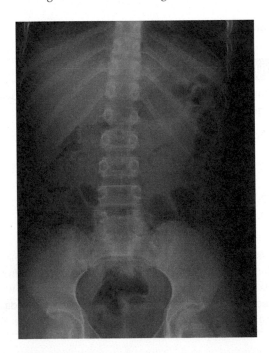

Figure 23.9 X-ray from the end of the second bowel management week.

Over the next six weeks, the child became defiant with rectal enemas and would not allow her mother to complete the administration. She started having trouble sleeping and began acting out and having trouble concentrating in school.

QUESTION 23.15

What could you offer this patient?

Answer: An antegrade flush option in conjuction with anal botulinum toxin to relax the anal sphincters was scheduled as the child had resolution of her abdominal and rectal pain with the rectal enemas.

The antegrade flush option and anal botulinum toxin were performed and the child was discharged home on her previous flush regimen of 500 mL of saline, 30 mL of glycerin, and 18 mL of Castile soap. The family reported the child was emptying well on the current regimen. There were occasional hard stools and smearing one to two times weekly.

Over the next months, the child had several antegrade regimen changes, oral medication changes, emergency department visits, and hospitalizations for hard stools, soiling, abdominal pain, nausea, vomiting, and rectal bleeding. The clinical team was concerned that the recommendations were not being adhered to.

QUESTION 23.16

What course of action would be recommended for this child?

A. Another bowel management week with antegrade flushes
B. Repeat motility testing
C. Inpatient bowel management
D. Stay the current course

Answer: It was recommended for the child to have inpatient bowel management to help assess compliance with the regimen/recommendations and determine a more successful and tolerable flush regimen (Answer C).

Figure 23.10 is the patient's X-ray at the beginning of inpatient bowel management.

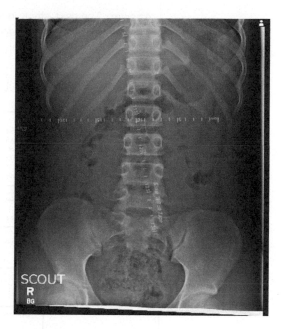

SCOUT
R
BG

Figure 23.10 X-ray from the first day of inpatient bowel management week.

QUESTION 23.17

What does the X-ray show? What would you do?

Answer: The X-ray shows a significant stool burden. A mineral oil rectal enema was given prior to the patient's flush of 600 mL of saline and 90 mL of glycerin to clean the rectum. This regimen caused significant cramping and nausea, therefore during days 2–4 of bowel management the glycerin was decreased to 60 mL and this eliminated the symptoms. Her stool output decreased over the course of several days. An exam under anesthesia found hard stool. A dose of 17 g of polyethylene glycol 3350 was added to the regimen twice daily. It became clear by the end of the third bowel management week that the patient was failing both antegrade flushes and rectal enemas and meets defecatory dysfunction criteria.

A patient with severe functional constipation, failed laxative treatment and both rectal and antegrade enemas

QUESTION 23.18

What would you do?

Answer: The next steps include repeating colonic manometry and plan for sacral nerve stimulator (SNS) evaluation for defecatory dysfunction criteria (see Figure 23.11) (Lu, 2017; Lu et al., 2018).

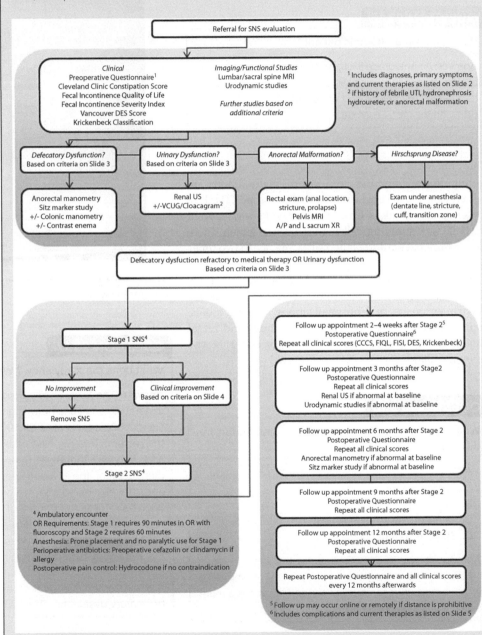

Figure 23.11 Sacral nerve stimulator evaluation protocol.

QUESTION 23.19

In the evaluation phase of the SNS protocol it is clear this patient has defecatory dysfunction. Which studies would you anticipate reviewing for this patient?

Answer: The studies you may review include anorectal manometry, sitz marker study, colonic manometry (optional), and contrast enema (optional). The information from these studies will help determine what may be contributing to her failed management and determine if she is a candidate for the SNS stage 1 trial. If the patient is a candidate for the trial and experiences improvement in symptoms, the patient should progress to stage 2 for her permanent SNS placement and ongoing follow-up.

This patient will also continue to follow urology for complaints of dysuria, incontinence, and urgency. She is encouraged to complete timed voiding every 2–3 hours whether she has the sensation to void or not. She has been instructed to double void with each trip to the toilet and continue pelvic floor relaxation with biofeedback exercises. The possible placement of the SNS may also benefit this patient's urinary symptoms by improving fecal burden.

KEY LEARNING POINTS

1. It must be determined if the patient's symptoms are related to constipation prior to considering any operative intervention such as an antegrade flush option.
2. If the child continues to have the same symptoms (abdominal and rectal pain) on rectal enemas, an antegrade option may not be indicated and further workup of their chronic abdominal pain is needed.
3. If the child has resolution of their abdominal and rectal pain with a successful rectal enema bowel management week, then an antegrade option would be the next course of action.
4. Botulinum toxin of the internal anal sphincter may be considered for the external anal sphincter

dyssynergia found during anorectal manometry, as it may assist in the relaxation of both sphincters and allow for easier passage of stool.

5. Consider anorectal biofeedback which utilizes neuromuscular conditioning techniques to treat patients with fecal incontinence or chronic constipation associated with dyssynergic constipation. Biofeedback is a tool to help patients learn how to perform muscle exercise training to relax the external anal sphincter and allow for easier passage of stool.
6. The rectal enemas were successful in this scenario but the antegrade flush option was not successful due to her pelvic floor dyssynergia. The rectal enema catheter helps keep the anal sphincters open and allow for evacuation of stool.
7. Inpatient bowel management may be necessary to assess compliance with the regimen and need for additional patient/family education.
8. An SNS is an option for defecatory dysfunction.
9. Urinary dysfunction is not uncommon in patients with defecatory dysfunction.

SUGGESTED READINGS

Lu, P. L. 2017. Sacral neuromodulation for constipation and fecal incontinence in children. *Seminars in Colon and Rectal Surgery*, 28, 185–188.

Lu, P. L., Koppen, I. J. N., Orsagh-Yentis, D. K. et al. 2018, February. Sacral nerve stimulation for constipation and fecal incontinence in children: Long-term outcomes, patient benefit, and parent satisfaction. *Neurogastroenterology & Motility*, 30(2). Retrieved from https://doi.org/10.1111/nmo.13184.

Wood, R. J., Yacob, D., & Levitt, M. A. 2016. Surgical options for the management of severe functional constipation in children. *Current Opinion Pediatrics*, 28, 370–379.

24

A patient who has recurrent constipation and soiling following colonic resection

ANDREA WAGNER

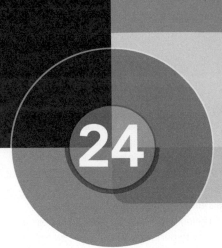

CASE HISTORY

A healthy 10-year-old female comes to your clinic with a history of functional constipation and daily fecal soiling. She passed meconium on the first day of life. She had a normal bowel movement pattern for her first 3 years. She developed constipation and soiling at age 4. She had previously tried the oral osmotic laxative Polyethylene glycol 3350 and sodium phosphate rectal enemas but had continued fecal soiling. She has no other past medical history, no significant urinary history, surgical history, family history, or social history.

In addition to normal anorectal physical exam findings, our initial evaluation of this patient included a contrast enema via the rectum (Figure 24.1).

Post-evacuation film is shown in (Figure 24.2).

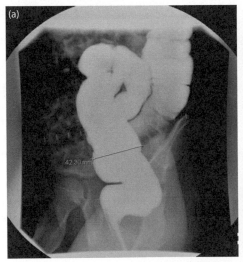 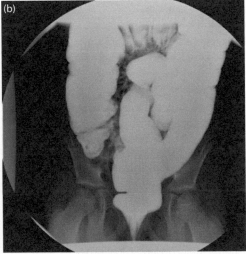

Figure 24.1 Contrast enema.

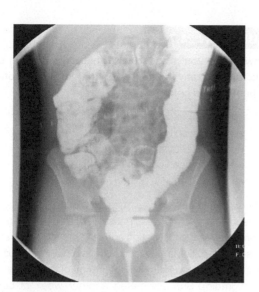

Figure 24.2 Past evacuation film.

QUESTION 24.1

How do you interpret the findings on the contrast enema?

Answer: The contrast enema shows a prominent ascending colon and a redundant and dilated sigmoid colon. These findings are consistent with chronic constipation. The dilation throughout suggests a slow moving or hypomotile colon.

QUESTION 24.2

What significant finding is revealed in the post evacuation image?

Answer: There is retained contrast on post-evacuation evaluation further supporting a slow moving or hypomotile colon.

This patient was started on a once daily dose (60 mg) of the oral stimulant laxative senna. The dose was administered once daily with the goal of producing one to two soft formed bowel movements per day. Her starting regimen was 60 mg senna once daily and 2 g of water-soluble fiber twice daily.

QUESTION 24.3

What is the goal of adding water-soluble fiber to this patient's daily laxative regimen?

Answer: The fiber will add bulk to her stool and make the laxative dose more effective, helping her to fully evacuate her rectum and distal sigmoid colon, preventing stool accumulation and resulting soiling.

The patient's report of the 24 hours following medication administration and her X-ray findings are as follows.

Patient report:

- Three large soft bowel movements 8–12 hours after laxative dose administration
  - The last bowel movement was less formed than the two prior
- Abdominal cramping and nausea
- Decreased food intake
- Soiling overnight (Figure 24.3)

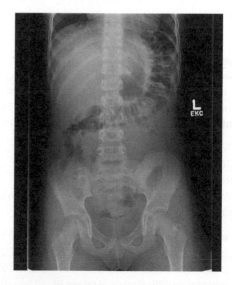

Figure 24.3 Abdominal X-ray.

QUESTION 24.4

What does this X-ray show with regard to stool volume?

Answer: There has been excellent stool evacuation with very little if any residual scattered stool throughout the colon. The patient has fully evacuated the contrast seen on the day prior to this X-ray.

QUESTION 24.5

What changes would you make to this patient's bowel regimen given the X-ray findings and her report of symptoms?

A. Increase laxative dose
B. Decrease laxative dose
C. Increase fiber dose
D. Decrease fiber dose

Answer: The decision was made to decrease the laxative dose based on the clean X-ray and patient's report of three large bowel movements and soiling overnight (Answer B). She also had symptoms of nausea and decreased oral intake, which could indicate a too-high laxative dose.

Her regimen at completion of bowel management week was 37.5 mg senna once daily and 2 g of water-soluble fiber twice daily. The patient's soiling was improved, but she continued to have accidents—two to three times per week.

QUESTION 24.6

What is your recommendation for this patient when you find she is having daily bowel movements, but has persistent soiling at the 3 month follow-up visit?

A. Colon resection
B. Gastroenterology (GI) referral for colonic and anorectal manometry
C. Malone appendicostomy for antegrade enema administration

Answer: Because this patient has failed the trial of medical management with her having continued soiling, the decision was made to refer the patient to GI for colonic and anorectal motility studies (Answer B).

- Anorectal manometry revealed normal pressures and intact rectoanal inhibitory reflex (RAIR).
- Colonic manometry testing revealed a good response to bisacodyl and glycerin with high amplitude propagating contractions (HAPCs) throughout the colon with exception of the last 35–40 cm.

QUESTION 24.7

How would you proceed with this patient given she has failed laxatives and has documented dysmotility in her sigmoid colon?

A. Malone appendicostomy for antegrade enema administration
B. Resection of dysmotile sigmoid colon and Malone appendicostomy for antegrade enema administration

Answer: The decision was made to proceed with Malone appendicostomy to provide patient with a trial of antegrade enemas to treat constipation and fecal soiling (Answer A). Most such patients respond well to antegrade flushes despite having a dysmotile segment of colon (usually the sigmoid). She completed another week of bowel management but despite many changes of the regimen over 3 months, was unable to find a Malone flush regimen that was effective at emptying her colon and that was well tolerated.

QUESTION 24.8

How would you proceed with this patient with a dysmotile sigmoid colon that has now failed oral stimulant laxatives and antegrade flushes via Malone appendicostomy?

Answer: The decision was made to proceed with resection of the dysmotile and redundant sigmoid colon. Post-resection, the patient did well with Malone flushes. She had 3 months of dramatically reduced fecal soiling (one to two episodes per month). However, four months post-resection she presented with nausea and vomiting after flush administration as well as worsening fecal soiling.

QUESTION 24.9

How would you evaluate this patient with clinical failure after colonic resection?

A. Abdominal X-ray
B. Change the flush ingredients
C. Repeat contrast study
D. All of the above

Answer: The decision was made to begin our investigation with an abdominal X-ray (Answer A).

Abdominal X-rays were obtained, which did not reveal a clear cause for nausea, vomiting or soiling (Figure 24.4).

The flush stimulant was then changed from glycerin to Castile soap without improvement, and Castile soap to bisacodyl without improvement. The decision was then made to proceed with a contrast study via the Malone appendicostomy.

Based on the concern for an anastomotic stricture seen in Figure 24.5, the decision was made to proceed with colonoscopy. The scope could not traverse a stricture found at about 8–10 cm from the anal verge. This area was balloon dilated and the scope then passed easily. Post-dilation, the patient was resumed on her initial post-resection regimen and tolerated this very well.

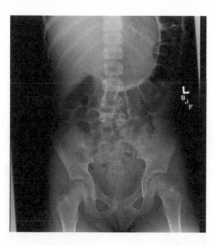

Figure 24.4 Abdominal X-ray.

QUESTION 24.10

What finding on this contrast study could explain flush intolerance and soiling after sigmoid resection and Malone placement (Figure 24.5)?

Answer: The answer is possible anastomotic stricture.

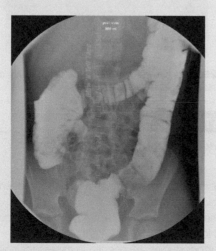

Figure 24.5 Contrast study.

QUESTION 24.11

If colonoscopy in this scenario had been normal and no anatomic concern was found, what steps might you consider next to continue your evaluation and treatment of a patient with persistent constipation and soiling, post-colonic resection?

    A. Repeat colonic manometry testing
    B. Consider placement of sacral nerve stimulator

Answer: Consider repeating colonic manometry testing (Answer A).

KEY LEARNING POINTS

1. Abnormal colonic motility can guide surgical resection when a patient has failed oral medical management and has a redundant sigmoid on contrast enema evaluation.
2. Most patients do well with antegrade flushes despite having a dysmotile colonic segment.
3. Contrast enema evaluation post-resection can reveal anatomic problems contributing to a patient's symptoms of persistent fecal soiling, especially if fecal soiling had initially reduced dramatically post-resection. The key exam is to simulate the flush with a contrast study via the Malone.
4. If a patient is struggling post-resection with persistent fecal soiling and an anatomic abnormality is not found, other options for evaluation and treatment include repeat colonic motility testing and evaluation for sacral nerve stimulator (SNS) placement.

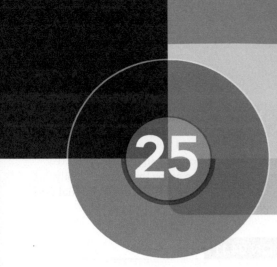
A young adult with intractable constipation and diffuse colonic dysmotility

ALESSANDRA GASIOR AND AMBER TRAUGOTT

CASE STUDY

A 28-year-old female presents with a history of constipation. Her symptoms also include bloating, abdominal pain, and the sensation of incomplete rectal emptying. She has one bowel movement every 2–3 weeks and denies any history of fecal incontinence. Her current medications include: lubiprostone (Amitiza®), linaclotide (Linzess®), polyethylene glycol 3350 (MiraLAX®), and polycarbophil (FiberCon®). In the past, she has trialed biofeedback for 2 months without any improvement.

On physical exam, the anorectal exam shows normal resting and squeeze tone with normal relaxation with Valsalva.

REVIEW MULTIPLE CHOICE QUESTIONS

QUESTION 25.1

What is your management plan for this patient?

A. Obtain anorectal manometry
B. Perform sitz marker study
C. Trial biofeedback
D. All of the above

Answer: D. Anorectal manometry is necessary to evaluate evacuatory function, a sitz marker test is used to evaluate colonic inertia, and biofeedback is useful to assess for improvement with pelvic floor physical therapy. A 2-month period typically is an insufficient time period to assess for treatment success.

The evaluation is performed and the results are shown in Figure 25.1.

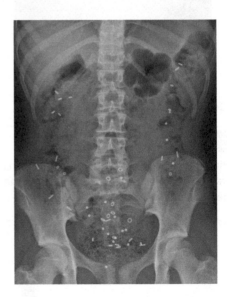

Figure 25.1 Abdominal film with sitz marker study on day #5 after ingestion of sitz markers.

QUESTION 25.2

What does the sitz marker study show?

A. Study shows diffuse colonic intertia
B. Sitz markers remaining show a normal pattern of colonic motility
C. The sigmoid represents the dysmotile portion of the colon
D. Further studies are needed to assess the colonic motility

Answer: A. More than 20% of the sitz markers remain in the colon, distributed from ascending colon to rectum, demonstrating diffuse colonic inertia.

Anorectal manometry is performed with the following results:

- Normal balloon expulsion test
- Avg resting pressure: 53.25 mmHg
- Avg squeeze pressures: 135.5 mmHg
- Positive rectal anal inhibitory reflex (RAIR)

QUESTION 25.3

What are the relevant findings from the anorectal manometry study?

A. Hirschsprung disease
B. Pelvic outlet dysfunction
C. Inadequate squeeze pressures
D. Normal pelvic floor function

Answer: D. The findings of normal balloon expulsion test rules out outlet dysfunction (also known as pelvic floor dyssynergia) and the presence of RAIR rules out Hirschsprung disease.

QUESTION 25.4

After reviewing the sitz marker study and anorectal manometry, how would you proceed?

A. Full-thickness rectal biopsy
B. Laparoscopic end ileostomy
C. Laparoscopic total abdominal colectomy with ileorectal anastomosis
D. Continue medical management for constipation

Answer: C. A laparoscopic total abdominal colectomy with ileorectal anastomosis is the most appropriate surgical procedure. An end ileostomy is more appropriate if the patient has significant pelvic floor dyssynergia. A full-thickness rectal biopsy would only be useful to rule out Hirschsprung disease, if the RAIR was negative on the anorectal manometry, and this diagnosis was suggested by the clinical history.

QUESTION 25.5

If the anorectal manometry showed an abnormal balloon expulsion (i.e., inability to push out balloon) how would this change your plan?

A. Full-thickness rectal biopsy
B. Laparoscopic total abdominal colectomy with end ileostomy
C. Laparoscopic total abdominal colectomy with ileorectal anastomosis, no change in plan
D. Pelvic floor physical therapy and biofeedback

Answer: D. If the patient is unable to expel the balloon on the anorectal manometry, then the patient has pelvic floor dyssynergia. A period of pelvic floor physical therapy, to include biofeedback, would be necessary. If this fails, the operative approach would be for a laparoscopic total abdominal colectomy with end ileostomy. Ileorectal anastomosis is not advised, because the functional outlet obstruction may increase the risk for anastomotic leak in the immediate postoperative period, owing to high pressure build-up in the rectum. Patients with outlet dysfunction and an ileorectal anastomosis have frequent liquid bowel movements (often 10–20 times per day) and rectal leakage.

KEY LEARNING POINTS

1. Initial evaluation should include sitz marker study to evaluate for colonic inertia.
2. Anorectal manometry should include a balloon expulsion test and evaluation for RAIR.
3. If RAIR is positive, this would rule out Hirschsprung disease.
4. The balloon expulsion test on the anorectal manometry demonstrates a negative workup for pelvic floor dyssynergia.
5. If the patient does not have pelvic floor dyssynergia, then a total abdominal colectomy with ileorectal anastomosis is the best surgical option.
6. If the patient has pelvic floor dyssynergia, a pelvic anastomosis would be ill-advised. Pelvic floor physical therapy and biofeedback should be performed prior to any operative intervention.

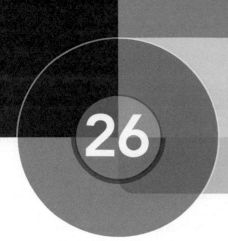
A young adult with pelvic floor dyssynergia

ALESSANDRA GASIOR AND AMBER TRAUGOTT

CASE STUDY

A 30-year-old female presents with a history of chronic constipation. She also complains of rectal pain with defecation. She has a history of multiple episodes of hospitalizations requiring disimpaction. She has progressive bloating worsened by laxatives. Her frequency of bowel movements are only one every few weeks, and to initiate them she must sit for long periods with multiple position adjustments and digital maneuvers to evacuate her rectum. Her current medications include: 8–10 laxatives per day (senna 86 mg) as well as linaclotide (Linzess®).

On physical exam, she has an anorectal exam with a hypertonic sphincter and absent relaxation with Valsalva.

QUESTION 26.1

What is the next step in the management of this patient?

A. Obtain anorectal manometry
B. Trial pelvic physical therapy and biofeedback
C. Order sitz marker study
D. All of the above

Answer: D. All of the above tests are necessary to fully evaluate the patient.

EVALUATION

The sitz marker study results are shown in Figure 26.1.

Sitz Marker Study with results shown after day 5 of ingestion of the sitz markers.

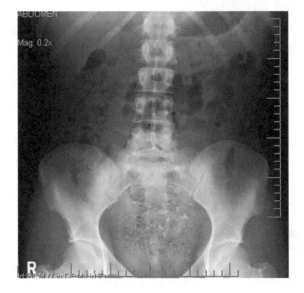

Figure 26.1 Abdominal X-ray with sitz markers.

QUESTION 26.2

What does the sitz marker study demonstrate after 5 days?

A. Diffuse colonic inertia
B. Pelvic outlet disorder
C. Segmental slow transit in descending colon only
D. Normal colonic motility

Answer: B. The sitz markers are all in the sigmoid colon and rectum and this coupled with a prolonged colonic transit time, demonstrating pelvic outlet dysfunction, or pelvic floor dyssynergia.

Anorectal manometry:

- Failure to pass balloon expulsion test
- Avg resting pressure: 80.1 mmHg
- Avg squeeze pressures: 148.1 mmHg
- Positive Rectal Anal Inhibitory Reflex

QUESTION 26.3

What do the anorectal manometry results tell you?

A. Diagnostic of Hirschsprung disease
B. Failure to pass the balloon expulsion test demonstrates pelvic floor dyssynergia
C. Normal anorectal manometry
D. Primary sphincter weakness

Answer: B. This anorectal manometry is abnormal as it shows failure to pass the balloon expulsion test, which is indicative for pelvic floor disorder. Hirschsprung disease can be ruled out as the rectoanal inhibitory reflex (RAIR) is positive. The sphincter pressures do not demonstrate weakness.

QUESTION 26.4

After reviewing the sitz marker study and the anorectal manometry findings, how would you proceed?

A. Full-thickness rectal biopsy
B. Refer patient to pelvic floor physical therapy and biofeedback
C. Laparoscopic loop colostomy
D. Laparoscopic total abdominal colectomy with ileorectal anastomosis

Answer: B. The sitz marker study does not demonstrate colonic inertia, but supports outlet dysfunction with the retained markers all within the rectosigmoid. The anorectal manometry also demonstrates pelvic floor dyssynergia. Therefore, the next step would be to refer this patient for pelvic floor physical therapy and biofeedback. Pelvic floor physical therapy serial treatments provides education on pelvic floor exercises to increase flexibility, stretch tight muscles, and strengthen weak ones. Biofeedback is a technique that can help patients see how their pelvic floor muscles are working.

QUESTION 26.5

If the patient fails to improve with pelvic floor physical therapy and biofeedback, what would you do next?

A. Total colectomy with end ileostomy
B. Loop colostomy without resection
C. A or B
D. Total abdominal colectomy with ileorectal anastomosis

Answer: C. If the patient fails pelvic floor physical therapy, the next best options for surgical management would be total colectomy with end ileostomy or loop colostomy without resection. A loop colostomy bypasses the functional pelvic floor obstruction, without the morbidity of an end ileostomy for long-term dehydration or electrolyte disturbances. Loop colostomy is only appropriate if colonic motility is relatively preserved.

KEY LEARNING POINTS

1. Based on her symptoms, physical exam findings, and evaluation, this patient has pelvic floor dyssynergia.
2. Colonic transit is considered abnormal if more than 5 sitz markers (20% retained) are present on plain abdominal film after 5 days.
3. Balloon expulsion test has an 80%–90% specificity, and 50% sensitivity for dyssnergia (Rao 2008).
4. Pelvic floor physical therapy with biofeedback has been shown to be superior to diazepam or placebo in treating pelvic floor dyssynergia (Heymen et al. 2007).

SUGGESTED READINGS

Heymen, S., Scarlett, Y., Jones, K. et al. 2007 April. Randomized, controlled trial shows biofeedback to be superior to alternative treatments for patients with pelvic floor dyssynergia-type constipation. *Diseases Colon Rectum*, 50(4), 428–441.

Rao, S. S. 2008 September. Dyssynergic defecation and biofeedback therapy. *Gastroenterology Clinics North America*, 37(3), 569–586.

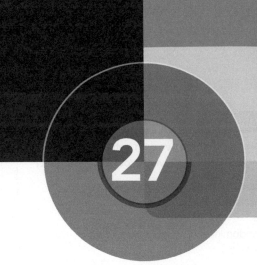

A patient with severe constipation and a behavioral disorder

KATRINA HALL, CHARAE KEYS, AND ROSE LUCEY SCHROEDL

27

CASE HISTORY

A 10-year-old child with functional constipation manifesting as soiling, bloating, and impaction beginning at the age of 2 presents for help with difficulty stooling. Many attempts at laxative treatments had failed in the past.

The patient was previously diagnosed with a mood disorder, sleep disturbance, Attention Deficit Hyperactivity Disorder (ADHD), Autism Spectrum Disorder, and disruptive behavior disorder. He has a history of atypical behaviors, including self-injury, chronic suicidal ideations, and hallucinations, and has been prescribed various medications to manage ADHD symptoms, stabilize his mood, and aid with sleep. The family disclosed a history of chronic physical and mental health conditions, in addition to barriers to resources and access to healthcare.

QUESTION 27.1

How would you manage this patient based on the social and medical information?

A. Do not consider the psychosocial aspects of the case in your plan of care.

B. Engage your psychosocial team members including psychology, child life, and social work at the start of the process.

C. Formulate a medical plan of care and engage your psychosocial team at the next follow –up visit.

D. Have the medical team make all assessments and consult psychology, child life, and social work only if they cannot solve the issue themselves.

Answer: B. Engaging the psychosocial team at time of initial evaluation will provide the medical team with psychosocial history that will benefit the multidisciplinary team regarding the patient's behavior, ability to complete the recommended regimen, assess for financial barriers to care, ability to cope with the regimen, and assess the parents' understanding of the medical recommendations. In an ideal situation, all team members meet the patient at the time of initial evaluation and then each team member utilizes their skills to provide the best care.

When the psychosocial team is utilized, they are able to advocate for the needs of patients and families, and influence decisions regarding the patient and family's medical needs, including their goals for treatment. Through their role and specific assessments, the psychosocial team is able to define what is achievable and realistic for families given their current regimen, the recommended regimen, and their environment outside of the hospital.

This child attended a week-long bowel management program and was started on a rectal enema regimen of 500 mL of saline and 30 mL of glycerin. A mechanical way to empty the colon was chosen because of prior failures with laxatives. During the initial visit, a behavior plan was created with the family for enema administration, including establishment of a routine, distraction, and contingency management with rewards and consequences for compliance. This plan encouraged the family to administer the enema at the same time each day as able, let the patient choose an activity of interest to engage in during the catheter insertion, and during the flush administration, and then allow the patient to identify high-saliency rewards for success, such as a treat or extra videogame time.

At the end of the week, the patient's X-ray showed that he was clean when enemas were successfully administered. However, uncooperative behavior required his caregivers to restrain him during enema administration.

QUESTION 27.2

What aspects of this child's history may have influenced his behavioral response to the enema administration?

A. Family history of chronic illness
B. Social history of abuse
C. Behavioral diagnoses
D. All of the above

Answer: D. Family history, behavioral diagnoses, and concerns regarding abuse/neglect should be discussed with the interdisciplinary team when considering a patient's regimen. It is also imperative to discuss with parents and guardians their ability to complete the enema administration, as they may have psychosocial history that prevents them from participating in their child's regimen.

QUESTION 27.3

After a child with behavioral problems and severe constipation has failed oral medication management and a trial of rectal enemas, what is your next course of action?

A. Surgical resection
B. Consider antegrade enemas
C. Inpatient bowel management

Answer: B. An antegrade enema regimen can promote independence and autonomy as the child can independently place the catheter in the channel created and administer the flush. The antegrade enema option can decrease the uncomfortable feeling many children complain of with rectal enema administration. The mechanical route is reliable and allows for "scheduling" of the daily stool, without concern for effects of laxatives such as nausea, cramping, or unexpected stooling.

QUESTION 27.4

What is this patient's best option for antegrade enema administration?

A. Cecostomy
B. Malone appendicostomy
C. Neomalone

Answer: A.

This is a challenging decision with multiple factors to consider. In this patient, the medical team chose to do a laparoscopic-assisted cecostomy for a few reasons:

1. Sometimes a thick abdominal wall can present difficulties for the surgeon where the native appendix cannot reach the umbilicus.
2. Some patients with behavioral and developmental needs may have difficulty with the sensory aspect and compliance of catheterization of the Malone site in the umbilicus. The ability to connect to an indwelling device can be less invasive for patients and promote cooperation.

Note: A Malone could also be created, and a device placed in it, so that the patient has both options, catheterization or leaving in an indwelling device.

After the patient attended the bowel management week, the medical team and family decided that an antegrade enema regimen would be the best option for the patient to aid with compliance.

The child was admitted a day prior to surgery to receive a preoperative bowel preparation with GoLYTELY through a nasogastric (NG) tube and intravenous (IV) fluids. The reason for this preoperative bowel preparation was because the patient was not on a reliable bowel regimen and he was regularly impacted. The multidisciplinary team determined a secure device would be a better option (instead of cathing), due to his behavioral and social history. Accessing the device is often less invasive for the patient, thus decreasing the risk of triggering trauma symptoms (i.e., defiance, aggressive behaviors). "Given that there is a direct preoperative anxiety to postoperative pain correlation for typically developing children, we must also consider the potential that heightened anxiety and maladaptive behaviors could produce a more challenging and painful post-operative experience for children with Autism Spectrum Disorder. It is the healthcare professional's responsibility to consider all issues when developing a plan of care for this patient population." (Wittling et al., 2018).

Antegrade flushes went well at first but two months later, the child came to the emergency department with a stool impaction.

QUESTION 27.5

What would you do first to relieve the child's stool impaction?

A. Prescribed flush through the Chait
B. GoLYTELY drip via cecostomy
C. Mineral oil enema
D. Manual disimpaction
E. Oral laxatives

Answer: B. GoLYTELY was started via the cecostomy; however, the child remained impacted. Then the psychosocial team influenced the decision to take the patient to the operating room (OR) for disimpaction rather than receiving enemas.

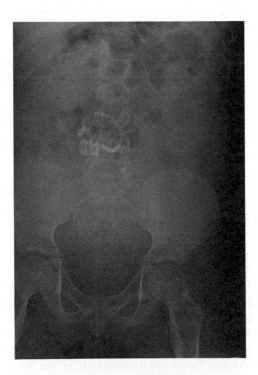

Figure 27.1 Patient's X-ray with stool burden.

After OR disimpaction, and continued GoLYTELY over several days, the colon was clean. After restarting a diet and daily flushes via the cecostomy, over the next few weeks he again became impacted. This occurred despite excellent compliance to the daily flush and increasing the flush concentration and volume (Figure 27.1).

The team felt a motility evaluation was needed due to the failure of medical management with laxatives, enemas, and antegrade flushes. The anorectal manometry (AMAN) was normal, demonstrating no sphincter dysfunction. A colonic manometry study (CMAN) showed that the patient's entire colon lacked the normal contractions to pass stool, which is also known as diffuse colonic dysmotility.

At this point it was decided to resect the majority of his dysmotile colon and leave him with only the right colon and access for a daily antegrade enema (his cecostomy). This was achieved via a subtotal colectomy with right colon to rectum anastomosis. The cecostomy remained in the right lower quadrant. In doing this, the child maintained antegrade access to flush the right colon and rectum. This approach gives the patient a chance to maintain a more normal "bowel movement pattern."

Postoperatively, the patient returned to the inpatient unit with a peripherally inserted central catheter (PICC) Foley, epidural for pain management, and nasogastric tube to suction. The patient's bowel function returned after 1 week. The patient's nil per os (NPO) status interrupted a normal routine, as the patient was unable to take their behavioral medications by mouth. The patient was in the hospital for a total of 22 days.

QUESTION 27.6

What would you do if a patient is unable to take behavioral medications by mouth?

A. Discontinue all behavioral health medications
B. Clonidine patch to assist with behavioral management
C. Consult psychology
D. Provide clonidine patch and psychology consult

Answer: B.

Interdisciplinary collaboration is essential for patients on a behavioral medication regimen to promote a smooth transition post operatively. Collaboration between the medical team, psychology, and pharmacology can promote better outcomes for the patient and reduce interruptions in the patient's routine. Since this patient was NPO, it was important to find ways to maintain the medical therapy similar to the patient's home medication regimen. The clonidine patch was a temporary option for the patient until he was able to start his usual behavioral medications by mouth.

Leading up to the final days of this patient's admission, the child became uncooperative with daily tasks. The patient displayed combative behavior towards the staff. A code was called by the staff due to the patient becoming combative after his mother left his bedside. The crisis team responded to the call and assisted staff in deescalating the patient.

QUESTION 27.7

What psychosocial team members should you consult now that this child and family are ready for discharge?

A. Nothing, up his medication
B. Psychology consult
C. Child life
D. Social work
E. B, C, and D

Answer: E. During the code, a child life specialist was present and able to redirect the child back to their room utilizing the child's interest in videogames. A behavior management plan was created to complete the required tasks with the child's interests being the reward for compliance with changing clothes, taking medications, and returning to his room. The social worker met with the family at his bedside to assess the needs and stressors related to ongoing admission, and also to provide counseling. Social work provided counseling regarding the family's ongoing stressors including the mother's own legal issues, health concerns, and overall impact of the hospitalization on the family unit.

Psychology was consulted on the day of discharge and developed a behavior plan to promote compliance with medication and oral intake. Consults to child life, psychology, and social work would ideally be made upon admission to the hospital when behavioral and familial concerns are identified. Interventions that allow the patient and family to have individualized care plans promote positive coping for the family unit, (Wittling et al., 2018).

This child continues to be seen in clinic for follow-up visits regarding their cecostomy flush regimen. Psychology continues to meet with the child, as his baseline behavior had not returned to how it was prior to hospitalizations, the explanation for which is thought to be related to medication titration. The child's last X-ray was shown to be clean, yet he was still having occasional accidents.

QUESTION 27.8

How would you manage this patient at this time?

A. Add laxatives to regimen
B. Add fiber to regimen
C. Add bisacodyl to flush regimen
D. Change flush to twice a day

Answer: B. Adding fiber to the patient's antegrade enema regimen will help bulk the stool. A child with only a small remaining segment of colon may experience liquid stool. Water-soluble fiber given throughout the day can add bulk to their stool, slowing overall motility, and decreasing occasional episodes of soiling.

KEY LEARNING POINTS

1. Antegrade enema options should be considered for patients with history of abuse and behavioral disorders as this option promotes independence and autonomy and avoid the rectal route.
2. A patient and family psychosocial history including past history of child abuse/neglect should be taken into consideration when prescribing a medical regimen.
3. Early involvement of the psychosocial team including child life, psychology, and social work can help patients, caregivers, and families address behavioral and psychiatric concerns to promote positive coping for patients and improve overall treatment response.
4. Patients with underlying behavioral concerns benefit from continuity of medication and behavioral interventions in the context of medical treatment to maintain gains of past behavioral health treatments, as well as aid with the recovery process.

SUGGESTED READING

Wittling, K., Dufur, J. P., McClain, A., & Gettis, M. 2018. Behavioral coping plans: One inter-professional team's approach to patient-centered care. *Journal of Pediatric Nursing*, 41, 135–139.

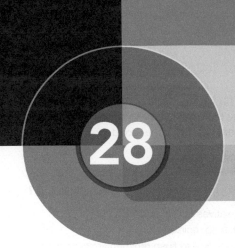

A young adult with incontinence after a low anterior resection

28

ALICIA FINN, SCOTT LAKE,
AND AMBER TRAUGOTT

CASE HISTORY

A 40-year-old female presents with fecal incontinence. She underwent neoadjuvant chemoradiation followed by low anterior resection for rectal cancer 5 years ago. She reports her incontinence started after surgery and has worsened since that time. She does not always feel the urge to defecate, and wears adult briefs daily both for passive stool leakage and for stool accidents. She has about four bowel movements per day, which are usually about an hour apart. They are sometimes loose in consistency. She has limited her activities outside the home, and carries extra clothes when she must go out in public. Her obstetric history includes two vaginal deliveries, which were only significant for an episiotomy with the second delivery.

Physical exam revealed very mild perianal skin thickening related to her prior radiation. Resting and squeeze tone were decreased on digital rectal examination. No mass or stricture was felt.

This patient had a Cleveland Clinic Incontinence Score of 15, indicating moderate to severe symptoms. Her FIQOL testing indicated her symptoms severely impacted the domains of lifestyle, coping, and embarrassment, while not correlating with symptoms of depression.

QUESTION 28.1

Which of the following instruments has been validated for evaluating fecal incontinence in adults?

A. Cleveland Clinic Incontinence Score (CCIS, also known as Wexner score)
B. Fecal Incontinence Quality of Life Scale (FIQOL)
C. Gastrointestinal Quality of Life Index (GIQLI)
D. Fecal Incontinence Severity Index (FISI)
E. All the above

Answer: E. Each of these instruments has been validated in adults with fecal incontinence. Selecting an appropriate instrument will depend on the context of the patient's symptoms, comorbidities, and type of treatment.

QUESTION 28.2

Which of the following diagnostic studies would *not* be indicated for her symptoms at this time?

A. Colonoscopy
B. CT of the abdomen and pelvis
C. Endorectal ultrasound
D. Anorectal manometry

Answer: B. Colonoscopy should be done to evaluate for pathologies that may contribute to her loose stools or incontinence. Endorectal ultrasound will evaluate for sphincter injury related to prior episiotomy. Anorectal manometry will evaluate defecatory mechanics, rectal sensitivity, and rectal compliance, any or all of which could be altered by prior rectal surgery and radiation. CT of the abdomen and pelvis would not be indicated.

QUESTION 28.3

What treatment recommendations can be made at the initial visit?

A. Increase fiber consumption
B. Trial pelvic floor physical therapy targeting sphincter strength and rectal sensation

C. Loperamide as needed for diarrhea

D. All of the above

Answer: D. Fiber bulks the stool, which can help to reduce diarrhea and to improve urge sensation and rectal emptying. Antidiarrheals such as loperamide can also help with loose stools. Pelvic floor physical therapy can improve neuromuscular function.

EVALUATION

Colonoscopy was performed and showed mild radiation-related changes in the remaining rectum and a healthy appearing colorectal anastomosis at 5 cm above the anal verge. The results were otherwise normal.

ANORECTAL MANOMETRY

- Resting sphincter pressure (mmHg): <20 mmHg
- Squeeze sphincter pressure (mmHg): 40 mmHg
- Positive rectal anal inhibitory reflex (RAIR)
- Threshold for first sensation (normal <20 mL): 40 mL
- Threshold for desire to defecate (normal 160–200 mL): 80 mL
- Passed balloon expulsion test

QUESTION 28.4

What do the anorectal manometry results tell you?

A. Primary sphincter weakness, normal rectal compliance and sensitivity

B. Primary sphincter weakness, decreased rectal compliance and sensitivity

C. Normal sphincter pressure, normal rectal compliance and sensitivity

D. Normal sphincter pressure, decreased rectal compliance and sensitivity

Answer: B. These results show weak resting and squeeze pressures. The elevated volume needed to feel first sensation shows decreased sensitivity. The lower volume needed to produce the desire to defecate indicates decreased rectal compliance. These findings are common after radiation and proctectomy for rectal cancer.

ENDOANAL ULTRASOUND

QUESTION 28.5

What does the endorectal ultrasound (EUS) show (Figure 28.1)?

A. Internal anal sphincter defect

B. External anal sphincter defect

C. Combined internal and external anal sphincter defect

D. No sphincter defect

Answer: D. The EUS shows that the internal and external sphincter muscles are both intact, though thin and atrophic.

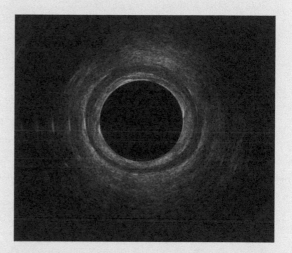

Figure 28.1 Endorectal ultrasound.

TREATMENT

QUESTION 28.6

This patient has multiple treatment options. Which of these would not be appropriate to offer this patient?

A. Sacral neuromodulation

B. Injectable anal canal bulking agents

C. Overlapping sphincteroplasty

D. Pelvic floor physical therapy alone

Answer: C. She is not a candidate for overlapping sphincteroplasty due to the results of the EUS, showing intact sphincters. Of the listed options, sacral neuromodulation and pelvic floor physical therapy have the greatest efficacy and durability of improvement in clinical trials.

After failing to achieve her goals with physical therapy, the patient underwent placement of a sacral neuromodulator. Her CCIS score decreased to 8 (mild symptoms) in subsequent visits, and her FIQOL scores improved to nearly normal in all domains at 3 months post-placement. She is able to be more active outside the home again and no longer wears adult diapers.

KEY LEARNING POINTS

1. Low anterior resection, with or without associated radiation treatment, can reduce sphincter tone and compliance and sensitivity of the rectum.
2. Initial management of fecal incontinence consists of bulking agents, antidiarrheals if needed, and pelvic floor physical therapy.
3. Subsequent treatment options may include sacral neuromodulation, injectable anal bulking agents, and/or overlapping sphincteroplasty as appropriate for the individual patient.
4. Multiple validated instruments can be used to evaluate patients with fecal incontinence and monitor their response to treatment.

SUGGESTED READINGS

Papaconstantinou, H. T. 2005. Evaluation of anal incontinence: Minimal approach, maximal effectiveness. *Clinics in Colon and Rectal Surgery*, 18(1), 9–16.

Ramage, L., Qiu, S., Kontovounisios, C., Tekkis, P., Rasheed, S., & Tan, E. 2015. A systematic review of sacral nerve stimulation for low anterior resection syndrome. *Colorectal Disease*, 17, 762–771.

Seong, M-K., Jung, S-I., Kim, T., & Joh, H-K. 2011. Comparative analysis of summary scoring systems in measuring fecal incontinence. *Journal of the Korean Surgical Society*, 81(5), 326–331.

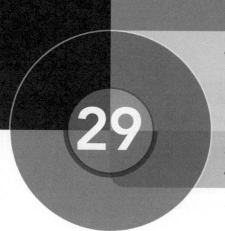

Two adults with incontinence after childbirth

29

STEPHANIE DOLAN, AMBER TRAUGOTT, AND POOJA ZAHORA

CASE HISTORY 1

A healthy 30-year-old female comes to your clinic with a history of fecal incontinence and incontinence to flatus for 3 years. She also complains of mild urinary stress incontinence for the last 6 months, for which she sees a urogynecologist. She states her bowel symptoms have been ongoing since the birth of her second child. She has had two live births, notable for third and fourth degree perineal lacerations, which were repaired at the time of delivery. The second child was her largest at 3.9 kg. She has bowel movements every 1–2 days and even when she does not have an accident she has symptoms of urgency. Her fecal incontinence episodes are about once per week and she has no control of flatus. She has bowel movements every 2–3 days. Her stool accidents interfere with her ability to engage in normal social activities. She has more severe symptoms with liquid stool than solid stool, but her stools are usually formed. She has been bulking her stool with fiber and it has helped somewhat. Her Cleveland Clinic Incontinence Score is 15. She had a colonoscopy 6 months ago, which was normal.

She has completed 16 weeks of pelvic floor physical therapy that has offered some improvement, but she and her physical therapist feel she has reached her plateau with this specific therapy. Her other medical history includes anxiety and gastroesophageal reflux disease (GERD). Her past surgical history includes a dilation and curettage postpartum as well as wisdom teeth extraction. She currently takes citalopram and lorazepam. Her social and family history are unremarkable.

On anorectal examination she has weak resting and squeeze tone and normal sphincter relaxation with Valsalva. She is also found to have a thin perineal body.

QUESTION 29.1

Which of the following is the most appropriate next step to evaluate this patient's treatment options for fecal incontinence?

- **A.** Pelvic magnetic resonance imaging (MRI)
- **B.** Sitz marker study
- **C.** Transrectal ultrasound
- **D.** CT of the abdomen and pelvis

Answer: C. Transrectal ultrasound can be used to evaluate whether a defect is present in the anal sphincter complex. This procedure can be performed in the office and does not require sedation. Obstetric trauma predisposes to sphincter injury, as well as possible pudendal nerve injury, both of which may contribute to fecal incontinence. Treatment options will differ if a sphincter defect is present.

The transrectal ultrasound findings are shown in Figure 29.1.

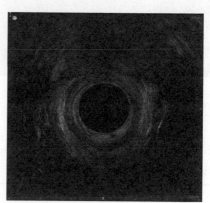

Figure 29.1 Transrectal ultrasound.

QUESTION 29.2

How do you interpret the findings on the transrectal ultrasound?

A. Normal
B. Posterior external anal sphincter defect measuring about 100 degrees
C. Anterior external anal sphincter defect measuring 100 degrees
D. Combined internal and external sphincter defect measuring 100 degrees

Answer: C. There is an anterior external anal sphincter defect measuring 100 degrees. On transrectal ultrasound, the internal anal sphincter typically has a darker or hypoechoic appearance. The external anal sphincter has a brighter appearance with more poorly defined borders. Normally, both sphincters will be circumferential without any defects seen (Figure 29.2).

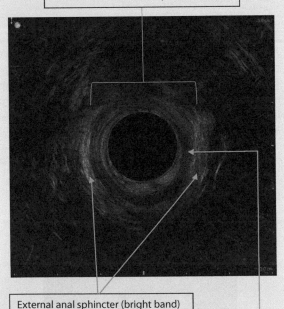

Anterior external anal sphincter defect

External anal sphincter (bright band)

Internal anal sphincter (dark band)

Figure 29.2 Transrectal ultrasound.

QUESTION 29.3

After considering the outcomes of her pelvic floor physical therapy and review of the transrectal ultrasound, which of the following options is most appropriate?

A. Continue pelvic floor physical therapy only
B. Sphincteroplasty with possible perineoplasty
C. Colostomy
D. Repeat colonoscopy

Answer: B. The best outcomes for sphincteroplasty are seen in young women after obstetric trauma. If other muscles of the perineum have been injured, a perineoplasty could be considered. This may be undertaken in combination with a specialist in female pelvic medicine and reconstructive surgery (urogynecology) if the patient has concomitant urinary symptoms. If there is no sphincter defect, the patient is not a candidate for sphincteroplasty. Sacral neuromodulation is an effective treatment for fecal and urinary incontinence, and is another appropriate option to discuss.

After discussion of risks, benefits, and alternatives, the decision was made to proceed with a sphincteroplasty, with possible perineoplasty as a combination case with urogynecology.

QUESTION 29.4

What are the major risks involved with this surgical procedure?

The major risks specific to the procedure include bleeding, infection, recurrent incontinence, injury to surrounding structures, and alteration of urinary or sexual function owing to nerve injury. Risks related to anesthesia may include cardiopulmonary complications, stroke, blood clots, and death, though these risks would be very unlikely in this patient.

QUESTION 29.5

What recovery restrictions will this patient have postoperatively?

Recovery restrictions include no heavy lifting greater than 10 pounds for 6 weeks, pelvic rest, and no sexual intercourse for 6 weeks.

Cleveland Clinic Incontinence Scale

Rarely = Less than once per month
Sometimes = At least once per month, but not every week
Usually = At least once per week, but not every day
Always = At least once per day

Symptoms	Frequency				
	Never	Rarely	Sometimes	Usually	Always
I do not have control of **solid** bowel movements	0	1	2	3	4
I do not have control of **liquid** bowel movements	0	1	2	3	4
I do not have control of **gas**	0	1	2	3	4
I wear a pad	0	1	2	3	4
I have had to make changes in my lifestyle because of my symptoms	0	1	2	3	4

Total score of 0 = perfect continence and 20 = total incontinence. The patient's score of 15 in the example reflects moderate to severe incontinence symptoms.

Figure 29.3 Cleveland clinic incontinence scale (Seong et al. 2011).

KEY LEARNING POINTS

1. Initial evaluation of fecal incontinence and sphincter defect should include an anorectal exam and transrectal ultrasound to evaluate the sphincters. Colonoscopy should be performed if this has not been done since the onset of symptoms.

2. Pelvic floor physical therapy is effective for many patients. It may obviate the need for surgery if the patient meets their treatment goals with physical therapy alone. A 4–6-month trial is reasonable before declaring failure of nonoperative management.

3. Surgical intervention with sphincteroplasty should be considered in young patients after obstetric trauma with a demonstrated sphincter defect. Older patients remote in time from their injury have poorer functional outcomes and a less durable improvement after this procedure, with more than half returning to baseline or worsened symptoms within 5 years.

4. Major risk factors for this surgical procedure include bleeding, infection, injury to surrounding structures, and alteration of urinary or sexual function owing to nerve injury.

CASE HISTORY 2

A 26-year-old female comes to your clinic with a history of fecal incontinence. She first started experiencing incontinence after childbirth where she had an episiotomy that resulted in a poorly healed perineal body. This has manifested as daily soiling. She has previously tried a constipating diet. With this, she is able to avoid many accidents; however, stools come in an unpredictable pattern. She has no other significant past medical history, surgical history, urinary history, family history, or social history.

QUESTION 29.6

After obtaining a history and physical what would you recommend in order to better assess this patient's perineal body?

A. Abdominal X-ray
B. Contrast enema
C. Pelvic exam in the clinic
D. Pelvic exam under anesthesia

Answer: B. At initial visit, the patient has a normal physical exam, with the exception of the anorectal region. The decision was made to perform this exam under anesthesia (Answer D). This allows use of electrical stimulation to determine the quality and location of the sphincters around the anus. Further imaging would not have provided information on the condition of the patient's perineal body.

The patient underwent an anorectal physical exam under anesthesia. During this exam, a normal posterior anus and dentate line was found (Figure 29.4).

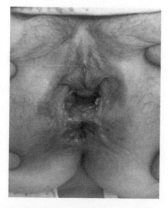

Figure 29.4 (See color insert.) EUA image of a disrupted perineal body.

The exam revealed a normal vagina and an absent perineal body. There was no sphincter palpable anterior to the anus, and it felt as if the muscles were lateral, indicating that they were split and the anus was not fully surrounded by sphincters. The introitus were right next to each other.

QUESTION 29.7

Why would damage to the perineal body cause fecal incontinence?

The perineal body lies just above the anal sphincter complex, which includes the internal and external sphincters. Together, these sphincters play a role in the squeezing and resting pressure of the anal canal. In this case, the sphincters anterior to the anus were separated by the poor perineal body healing. Therefore, the patient lacked the ability to close the sphincter muscle and thus close the anus when stool passed.

QUESTION 29.8

After an anorectal physical exam such as this, what would be the next step in managing this patient? Are there any options for treatment other than surgery?

Due to the damage to the perineal body, the patient lacks the ability to close the sphincter muscles, thus she would not have good potential to be continent on laxatives as the muscles need repair. However, the use of enemas could be considered, but this would mean the patient would have to complete lifelong enemas daily.

In repairing the perineal muscles, this would give the patient good potential for continence, given the muscles lying adjacent to the perineal body would be brought together.

The decision was made to proceed with surgical intervention and the patient underwent perineal body reconstruction to bring the sphincter muscles back together in order to have proper anatomy for bowel continence.

During the surgery, the perineal body muscle and the perineal body skin were reconstructed after mobilizing the anterior rectal wall. This technique is nearly identical to the one used in girls who undergo a redo for a dehisced perineal body after anorectal malformation repair. After this reconstruction was completed, the anterior rectal wall was resutured to the skin. The plan following surgery was another anorectal exam in 1 month.

Of note, it was advised by her obstetrician/gynecologist to have her second child via a vaginal delivery prior to this perineal body reconstruction, noting that once the perineal body was reconstructed, future deliveries would need to be by cesarean section.

At 1 month follow-up, the patient was doing well, with improved pain. At this time she reported being continent for stool. The exam revealed that the perineal body was well healed and was now 2–3 cm in length.

QUESTION 29.9

What discharge instructions would you provide to this patient?

The patient was instructed to wait before starting sexual activity for 3 months and to follow up with her obstetrician/gynecologist for contraceptive needs. She was instructed to return as needed for follow-up.

KEY LEARNING POINTS

1. Due to the close relationship between the perineal body and anal sphincter complex, damage to the perineal body can cause fecal incontinence.
2. In a female with fecal incontinence post-childbirth, examination of anatomy is key.
3. Reconstruction of the perineal body brings the muscles back together anterior to the anus.
4. This scenario is commonly seen in children who suffer from a perineal body dehiscence after a posterior sagittal anorectoplasty for imperforated anus.

SUGGESTED READINGS

Bravo Gutierrez, A., Madoff, R. D., Lowry, A. C., Parker, S. C., Buie, W. D., & Baxter, N. N. 2004. Long-term results of anterior sphincteroplasty. *Diseases of the Colon and Rectum* 47, 727–732.

Duelund-Jakobsen, J., Worsoe, J., Lundby, L., Christensen, P., & Krogh, K. 2016. Management of patient with fecal incontinence. *Therapeutic Advances in Gastroenterology*, 8(1), 86–97.

Meyer, I. & Richter, H. E. 2016. Evidence-based update on treatments for fecal incontinence in women. *Obstetrics and Gynecology Clinics of North America*, 43(1), 93–119.

Oom, D. M., Gosselink, M. P., & Schouten, W. R. 2009. Anterior sphincteroplasty for fecal incontinence: a single center experience in the era of sacral neuromodulation. *Diseases of the Colon and Rectum*, 52, 1681–1687.

Seong, M. K., Jung, S. I., Kim, T., & Joh, H. K. 2011. Comparative analysis of summary scoring systems in measuring fecal incontinence. *Journal of the Korean Surgical Society* 81(5), 326–331.

Zorcolo, L., Covotta, L., & Bartolo, D. C. 2005. Outcome of anterior sphincter repair for obstetric injury: comparison of early and late results. *Diseases of the Colon and Rectum* 48, 524–531.

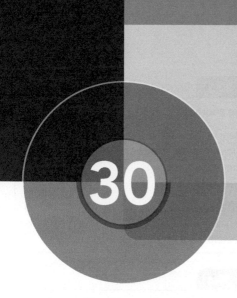

30

A young adult with rectal pain and fecal urgency who is a candidate for sacral nerve stimulation

ALESSANDRA GASIOR AND AMBER TRAUGOTT

A 28-year-old female presents with a history of rectal pain and fecal urgency. She has had three vaginal deliveries without significant obstetric trauma. She describes an "electric" type of rectal pain that comes and goes. She will suddenly have an urge to have a bowel movement and will barely make it to the restroom. She has fecal incontinence with soiling several times per week. Currently, she is taking glycerin suppositories as needed.

On physical exam, a digital rectal exam reveals no masses or tenderness. The resting sphincter tone is decreased. There is no appreciable squeeze on Valsalva.

QUESTION 30.1

What would be your next step in management?

A. Perform an endorectal ultrasound (EUS)
B. Obtain anorectal manometry
C. Refer patient to pelvic floor physical therapy and biofeedback
D. All of the above

Answer: D. All of the above are necessary to complete the workup for fecal incontinence.

An EUS allows examination of the internal and external sphincter complex to evaluate the integrity of the muscles. Anorectal manometry shows the functionality of these muscles and the ability to empty the rectum. Pelvic floor physical therapy allows the patient to work with a certified physical therapist to regain functionality of the pelvic floor.

EVALUATIONS

The EUS results are shown in Figures 30.1 and 30.2.

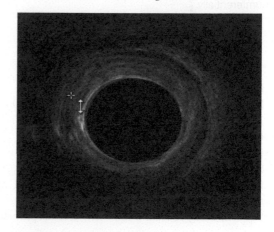

Figure 30.1 Anorectal ultrasound.

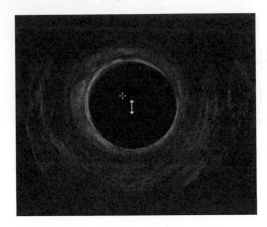

Figure 30.2 Anorectal ultrasound.

What does the anorectal manometry study tell you?

- **A.** Incompetent internal and external sphincters
- **B.** Concern for pelvic outlet disorder
- **C.** Incomplete rectal emptying
- **D.** All of the above

Answer: D. The anorectal manometry demonstrates pelvic floor disorder with inability to expel the balloon as well as incompetent internal and external sphincters.

Given these imaging findings, what would be the next best course of action for this patient?

- **A.** Continued pelvic floor physical therapy and biofeedback
- **B.** Full-thickness rectal biopsy
- **C.** Laparoscopic end ileostomy
- **D.** Sacral neuromodulation

Answer: A. With EUS demonstrating intact sphincters and anorectal manometry showing pelvic floor dysfunction, the next course of action would be pelvic floor physical therapy and biofeedback.

What does the endorectal ultrasound show?

- **A.** Internal anal sphincter with anterior defect
- **B.** External anal sphincter with posterior defect
- **C.** Intact internal and external anal sphincters
- **D.** A and B

Answer: C. The EUS shows that the internal and external sphincters are both intact; however, they are atrophic as you can see a thinning of the muscle complex circumferentially.

The anorectal manometry results were as follows:

- Rectoanal inhibitory reflex (RAIR) present
- Maximum tolerable volume: (normal >200 mL): 200 mL
- Unable to expel balloon
- Resting sphincter pressure: 3 mm Hg
- Squeeze sphincter pressure: <10 mm Hg
- Resting study reveals incompetent internal anal sphincter secondary to low resting pressure
- Squeeze study reveals weak external anal sphincter

Although she has made some progress, your patient continues to have issues with stool urgency and difficulty evacuating, despite pelvic floor physical therapy and biofeedback. What would you offer next?

- **A.** Continued pelvic floor physical therapy and biofeedback
- **B.** Two-week trial with sacral neuromodulation with a temporary power source to gauge its effectiveness prior to placement of a permanent device
- **C.** Laparoscopic end ileostomy
- **D.** Laparoscopic loop colostomy

Answer: B. If pelvic physical therapy fails, a trial of a sacral neuromodulation placement can be helpful with an overall success rate of 60%–80% in the limited studies available (Leroi et al., 2005).

After a two-week trial that demonstrates improvements in symptomatology with a temporary sacral nerve stimulator, a permanent neuromodulator may be placed.

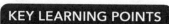

KEY LEARNING POINTS

1. The endorectal ultrasound shows atrophic but intact sphincters.
2. The anorectal manometry demonstrates incompetent internal and external sphincters, elevated sensation threshold, and inability to expel the balloon.

SUGGESTED READING

Leroi, A. M., Parc, Y., Lehur, P. A. et al. 2005. Efficacy of sacral nerve stimulation for fecal incontinence: Results of a multicenter double-blind crossover study. *Annals of Surgery* 242, 662–669.

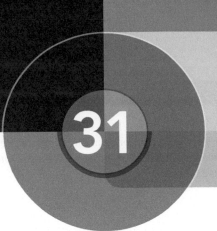

An adult with soiling following an ileoanal pouch

31

ALICIA FINN AND AMBER TRAUGOTT

CASE HISTORY

A 25-year-old male with a past medical history significant for ulcerative colitis previously underwent a three-stage restorative proctocolectomy with ileal pouch–anal anastomosis (J pouch). One month after his temporary ileostomy reversal, he comes to the office for his routine postoperative visit. He reports having 8–12 nonbloody bowel movements per day and this is causing his perianal skin to feel "raw." He is having leakage of liquid stool, especially at night. On examination, his perianal skin is red and excoriated, and he cannot tolerate a digital rectal exam.

The patient did well for many months using loperamide and fiber supplementation, and achieved a new baseline frequency of 4–5 bowel movements daily without seepage. He returns after 6 months because he has new pelvic pain and has had an increase in his bowel movement frequency from 4–5 times to 6–10 times daily for the past 2 weeks. He had stopped having seepage on loperamide and fiber, but now is having recurrent leakage which requires him to wear a pad in his clothes. He denies hematochezia, urinary urgency or frequency, fevers, or nausea and vomiting. He denies being on recent antibiotics, which may have altered the normal bacterial flora of the intestine. On physical examination, his abdomen is soft

and nontender. Digital rectal examination, now tolerable compared to initial presentation, reveals some mild stenosis at the anastomosis and mild tenderness without gross blood.

QUESTION 31.1

What is the most likely reason he is having stools at this frequency?

A. *Clostridium difficile* infection
B. Pouchitis
C. Viral gastroenteritis
D. Normal ileal pouch function

Answer: When continuity is initially established, patients with an ileal pouch–anal anastomosis (J pouch) are expected to have 8–10 bowel movements daily (Answer D). The ileal pouch does not have the same capacity to hold stool as a normal rectum and the mucosa are adjusting to having feces pass through; therefore, its contents are more liquid and more frequent. Typically, over a 6–12-month period, the reservoir stretches and adapts, sphincters strengthen, and the bowels start to absorb more water, which will thicken the stool and allow for better control. Patients typically average 4–8 bowel movements daily, even after adaptation.

QUESTION 31.2

Which of the following would be appropriate to prescribe to the patient at this time?

A. Loperamide
B. Fiber supplement
C. Barrier cream to perianal skin
D. All of the above

Answer: Antidiarrheals and fiber supplementation will help bulk the stool and reduce the frequency of bowel movements. Application of a perianal barrier cream will help the skin to heal and prevent further skin breakdown (Answer D). The ointments below are all used as first-line barriers. Choice depends on goals of therapy, individual preference, and ease of availability (Table 31.1).

Table 31.1 Types of perianal barrier cream

Product	Active ingredient	Advantages	Availability	Prescription needed
Desitin Maximum Strength	Zinc oxide (40%)	Provides thick protective moisture barrier	Available in stores and online	No
Critic-Aid Clear	Petrolatum (71.5%)	Provides clear moisture barrier. Allows for easy assessment of area. Able to apply to moist skin	Available online but is a special order at the pharmacy	No
Calmoseptine	Menthol (0.44%), Zinc oxide (20.6%)	Provides protective moisture barrier. Cooling and soothing properties	Available in stores and online	No

QUESTION 31.3

What would be your most likely diagnosis?

A. *Clostridium difficile* infection
B. Pouchitis
C. Viral gastroenteritis
D. Urinary tract infection

Answer: In the absence of fevers, nausea, vomiting, or urinary symptoms, the most likely cause for pelvic pain and increased stool frequency in a patient with an ileal pouch is pouchitis (Answer B). Pouchitis is an inflammation of the ileal pouch. Its etiology is not clearly known, but it is thought to result from an immune response to the gut microflora within the pouch.

QUESTION 31.4

Which of the following tests would confirm the diagnosis of pouchitis?

A. Complete blood count (CBC) with differential
B. Stool infectious studies
C. C-reactive protein (CRP) level
D. Colonoscopy
E. Pouchoscopy

Answer: Pouchitis is diagnosed by endoscopic visualization of the pouch and biopsies of the mucosa (Answer E). Biopsies typically show mild to severe inflammation, patchy or diffuse, and ulcers and/or erosions. Pouchoscopy is the correct term for endoscopic evaluation of an ileal pouch. Colonoscopy would not be the appropriate term because this patient's colon has been previously removed. Stool studies may be appropriate to rule out intestinal infectious pathogens, but would not confirm pouchitis. A CBC would not give useful information. CRP is a nonspecific inflammatory marker that could be elevated due to any infectious or inflammatory condition, and is not specific for pouchitis, if abnormal.

A pouchoscopy was performed (Figure 31.1).

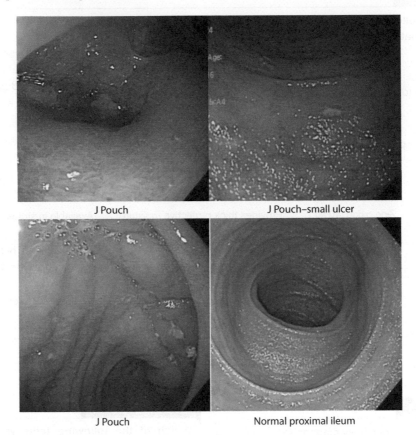

Figure 31.1 (**See color insert.**) Pouchoscopy images.

QUESTION 31.5

What is your opinion of how the pouch looked?

Answer: Mild inflammation is seen in the ileoanal pouch with a small aphthous ulcer. Biopsy was positive for mild patchy acute enteritis, favoring pouchitis.

QUESTION 31.6

Which of the following is *not* appropriate for the medical management of pouchitis?

A. Probiotic
B. Vancomycin enemas
C. Ciprofloxacin
D. Metronidazole

Answer: Treatment of pouchitis focuses on manipulating the gastrointestinal flora to reduce the inflammatory response. There is clinical evidence to support the use of probiotics, ciprofloxacin, and metronidazole for the treatment of pouchitis (Answer B).

The patient was placed on a probiotic for 6 weeks and his symptoms improved, but did not resolve. He was then placed on a 3-week course of ciprofloxacin with resolution of symptoms. Bowel movements decreased to 4–6 times a day and pelvic pain and seepage resolved.

KEY LEARNING POINTS

1. Liquid stool is a major contributor to seepage in patients with ileal pouch–anal anastomosis. Antidiarrheals such as loperamide can be used to thicken the consistency of the stool. Fiber supplementation can also bulk the stool and reduce seepage.

2. Pouchitis is a common inflammatory condition of the ileal reservoir of an ileal pouch–anal anastomosis. It seems to be an inappropriate immune response to the intestinal flora.

3. Some common symptoms of pouchitis are abdominal cramps, increased stool frequency and urgency, pelvic pressure, and tenesmus.

4. Pouchitis is treated with probiotics or selected antibiotics. Uncommonly, patients may require long-term antibiotic treatment to achieve remission of their symptoms.

SUGGESTED READINGS

Gionchetti, P., Calabrese, C., Lauri, A., & Rizzello, F. 2015. The therapeutic potential of antibiotics and probiotics in the treatment of pouchitis. *Expert Review of Gastroenterology and Hepatology,* 9(9), 1175–1181.

Lichtenstein, L., Avni-Biron, I., & Ben-Bassat, O. 2016. The current place of probiotics and prebiotics in the treatment of pouchitis. *Best Practice & Research Clinical Gastroenterology,* 30(1), 73–80.

Michelassi, F., Lee, J., Rubin, M., Fichera, A., Kasza, K., Karrison, T., & Hurst, R. D. 2003. Long-term functional results after ileal pouch anal restorative proctocolectomy for ulcerative colitis: A prospective observational study. *Annals of Surgery,* 238(3), 433–441.

PART

VI

RADIOLOGY

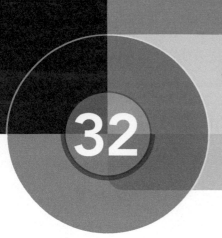

Which X-ray is worse?

32

ONNALISA NASH

In the management of fecal incontinence, abdominal X-rays are very helpful objective assessors of stool content. Based on this, the bowel regimen is altered for the desired effect. In this chapter you will see two X-rays, side by side, and need to determine which X-ray shows more stool in the colon.

QUESTION 32.2

Which X-ray has more stool throughout, A or B (Figure 32.2)?

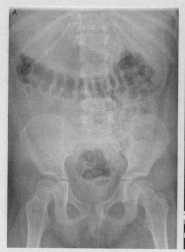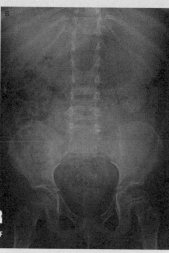

Figure 32.2 Abdominal X-rays.

Answer: B.

QUESTION 32.3

Which X-ray has more stool throughout, A or B (Figure 32.3)?

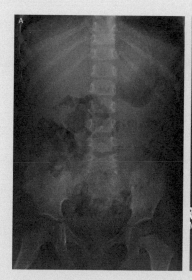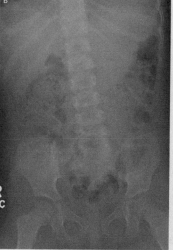

Figure 32.3 Abdominal X-rays.

Answer: A.

QUESTION 32.4

Which X-ray is concerning for possible bowel obstruction, A or B (Figure 32.4)?

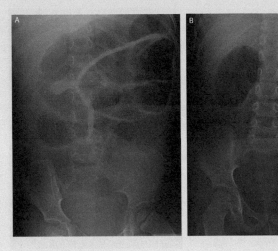

Figure 32.4 Abdominal X-rays.

Answer: A.

QUESTION 32.5

Which X-ray reveals an effective flush regimen, A or B (Figure 32.5)?

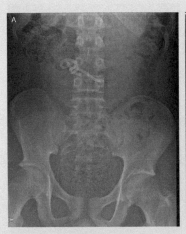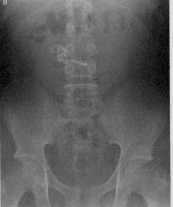

Figure 32.5 Abdominal X-rays.

Answer: B.

QUESTION 32.6

Which X-ray is worse, A or B (Figure 32.6)?

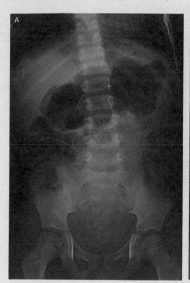
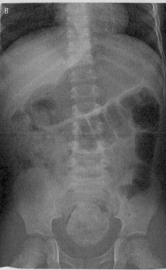

Figure 32.6 Abdominal X-rays.

Answer: B.

QUESTION 32.7

Which X-ray has more stool, A or B (Figure 32.7)?

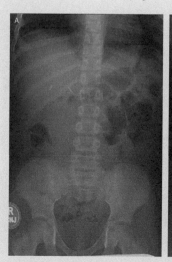
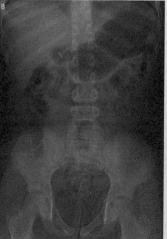

Figure 32.7 Abdominal X-rays.

Answer: A.

QUESTION 32.8

Which X-ray is worse, A or B (Figure 32.8)?

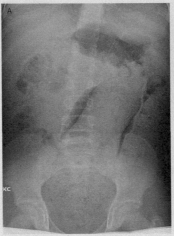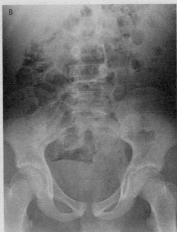

Figure 32.8 Abdominal X-rays.

Answer: A.

QUESTION 32.9

Which X-ray reveals more stool, A or B (Figure 32.9)?

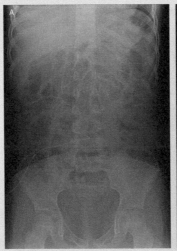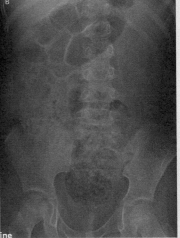

Figure 32.9 Abdominal X-rays.

Answer: B.

QUESTION 32.10

Which X-ray reveals less stool, A or B (Figure 32.10)?

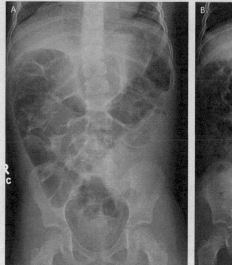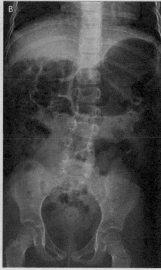

Figure 32.10 Abdominal X-rays.

Answer: A.

Interesting radiological findings

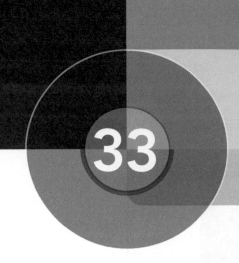

ONNALISA NASH AND MARC A. LEVITT

Imaging is frequently obtained for colorectal patients throughout their treatment to help guide surgical planning and bowel management. Often, radiological imaging reveals interesting information regarding the patient's anatomy that can have important implications on their management. This chapter includes several examples of these types of radiological findings. Throughout the chapter, we will ask what you perceive from the images.

QUESTION 33.1

What is an interesting finding in the image shown in Figure 33.1, of the colon of a 4-year-old male with a history of anorectal malformation (ARM)?

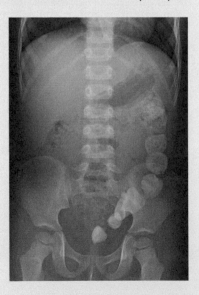

Figure 33.1 Contrast enema of 4yo male with ARM.

Answer: The child had a pull-through of his sigmoid colon as there is no rectum noted on the contrast study and one can see haustration in the pelvis. This means the rectum was previously removed (through an old-fashioned operation called an abdominoperineal pull-through). One can expect hypermotility in such a case and the need for a mechanical emptying process, because without a normal anal canal (as occurs in a patient with an ARM) and deficient sphincters, and hypermotility induced by the loss of the rectal reservoir, one cannot expect the patient to have voluntary bowel control.

QUESTION 33.2

With the following contrast study of a 6-year-old with Hirschsprung disease (HD), would you predict the child's original transition zone was proximal or distal to the splenic flexure (Figure 33.2)?

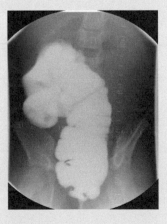

Figure 33.2 Contrast enema of 6yo with HD.

Answer: The contrast study reveals what appears to be a right-sided pull-through, which would indicate an original transition zone at the hepatic flexure. The right colon was all the ganglionated bowel that the patient had. One can expect hypermotility in such a case.

QUESTION 33.3

In regard to the image in Figure 33.3 of a 6-year old male with functional constipation (FC) and soiling, would you recommend a laxative regimen or a mechanical (enema) regimen?

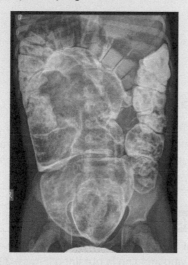

Figure 33.3 Contrast enema of 6yo with FC.

Answer: This contrast study reveals an extremely dilated rectosigmoid and the patient will more than likely need a mechanical regimen to empty, at least to start. Given this amount of dilation, laxatives will not work well to empty the colon and will cause significant cramping. Enemas may also not work and thus a motility evaluation including anorectal and possible colonic manometry will be needed to guide further therapy.

QUESTION 33.4

The image in Figure 33.4 was obtained from a patient in the immediate postoperative period after a redo posterior sagittal anorectoplasty (PSARP). The patient starts to have abdominal distension, nausea, and vomiting. What is your assessment and explanation for the symptoms?

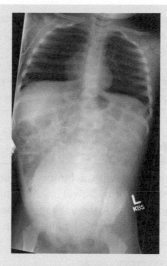

Figure 33.4 Abdominal X-ray after redo PSARP.

Answer: The X-ray reveals a pelvic cystic structure—it is the patient's large distended bladder. This dilated bladder, due to urinary retention, can compress the colon and cause these symptoms. Decompression of the bladder led to resolution of the problem.

QUESTION 33.5

A 2-year-old male with a history of Hirschsprung disease, who underwent a Soave pull-through as a newborn, presents with obstructive symptoms (distension and difficulty emptying) with several episodes of enterocolitis. The following imaging is obtained (Figure 33.5). What is a possible cause for the obstruction based on the imaging?

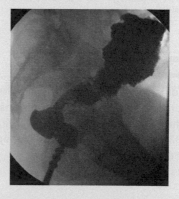

Figure 33.5 Contrast enema of 2yo male with HD and obstructive symptoms.

Answer: The image reveals a widened presacral space, which in the presence of a Soave pull-through is indicative of an obstructing Soave cuff. It is likely that the cuff was never adequately split, fused back together, or rolled up, leading to an external compression of the pull-through. The treatment for this is to surgically remove the cuff.

QUESTION 33.6

A 4-year-old male with a history of Hirschsprung disease presents for bowel management due to difficulty emptying. After assessing the images in Figure 33.6, which type of pull-through would you presume the patient had?

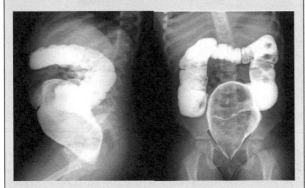

Figure 33.6 Contrast enema of 4yo with HD.

Answer: The imaging is most suggestive of a Duhamel technique with the ganglionated bowel stapled to the native rectum. The pouch is enormous, will be difficult to empty, and may need to be surgically removed during a redo operation.

QUESTION 33.7

A 2-year-old female with a history of Hirschsprung disease presents with abdominal distension, fever, and diarrhea. After assessing the following imaging (Figure 33.7), what specific finding supports a diagnosis of enterocolitis?

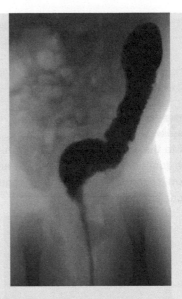

Figure 33.7 Contrast enema of 2yo with HD.

Answer: The jagged appearance of the descending colon is suggestive of enterocolitis. Ideally, a contrast enema should not be done during an episode of enterocolitis because perforation can occur.

QUESTION 33.8

A patient with an ARM presents for evaluation and the following imaging is obtained (Figure 33.8). What is concerning?

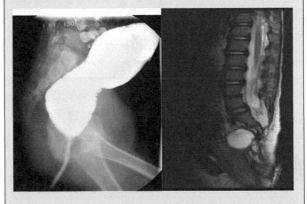

Figure 33.8 Contrast enema and MRI of patient with ARM.

Answer: The contrast enema reveals a widened presacral space, which in a patient with an ARM should make the clinician suspicious for a presacral mass. In this case, as seen on MRI, this correlated with a mass that was resected and turned out to be a teratoma. This situation must be particularly suspected in ARM patients with anal stenosis or rectal atresia.

QUESTION 33.9

A 2-year-old female with a history of ARM and tethered cord came to the emergency department because she has not stooled for 48 hours and is refusing to eat. She is on 8.8 mg of senna daily and usually stools 3–4 times per day. The following image is obtained (Figure 33.9). What significant finding is noted on the X-ray?

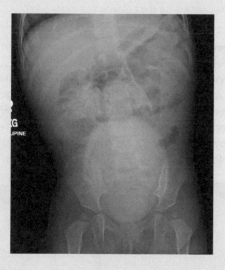

Figure 33.9 Abdominal X-ray of 2yo with ARM.

Answer: The bladder is grossly distended, indicating urinary retention, which is the likely cause of her constipation.

QUESTION 33.10

An 8-year-old female with a history of ARM is managed with cecostomy flushes. She has complaints of pain, nausea, and cramping during the flush with her current regimen. The following imaging is obtained (Figure 33.10). What interesting finding is causing the symptoms?

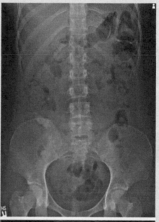

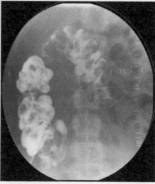

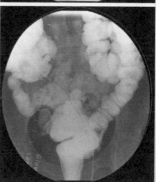

Figure 33.10 Contrast enema of 8yo with ARM.

Answer: The contrast study reveals retrograde flow of the contrast into the terminal ileum. The stimulants commonly used in flushes can cause these symptoms if the child has an incompetent ileocecal valve. The flush will likely be ineffective in emptying the colon as only a small amount of fluid enters the colon. Interventional radiology can place an extended tube into the right colon to alleviate these symptoms.

QUESTION 33.11

A 2-year-old presents with recurrent episodes of enterocolitis after their pull-through. What does this image represent (Figure 33.11)?

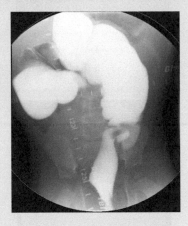

Figure 33.11 Contrast enema of 2yo with HD.

Answer: There appears to be a twist in the pull-through, which will need reoperative surgery to correct.

QUESTION 33.12

A 5-year-old male who underwent a redo pull-through for an obstructing Soave cuff and transition zone, protected by an ileostomy, then underwent ileostomy closure 3 months later. Now on postoperative day 3 he is vomiting. What is the diagnosis and treatment (Figure 33.12)?

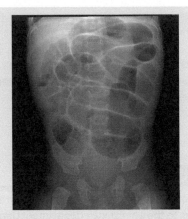

Figure 33.12 Abdominal X-ray of 5yo with HD.

Answer: The X-ray reveals dilated small bowel that is likely to be consistent with an ileus. A nasogastric tube will help relieve symptoms until the ileus resolves. Irrigations will not help this patient as the colon is not dilated.

QUESTION 33.13

A 10-year-old female with a history of cloaca presents for bowel management. Her current bowel regimen is Malone flushes. Her current symptoms are soiling and incomplete emptying with flushes. Her contrast enema is shown in Figure 33.13. What could be causing the symptoms?

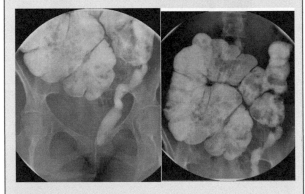

Figure 33.13 Contrast enema of 10yo with cloaca.

Answer: The contrast study reveals a stricture at the previous colostomy takedown site and narrowing of the distal pull-through segment. This has caused significant dilation of the proximal colon over time and is causing the current symptoms. This will need to be surgically repaired.

QUESTION 33.14

A 9-year-old boy presents for bowel management with a history of constipation and fecal soiling. What is an interesting finding on his contrast enema (Figure 33.14)?

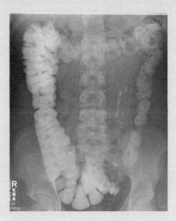

Figure 33.14 Contrast enema of 9yo with FC.

Answer: The contrast enema reveals that the cecum falls into the pelvis. If one did not know this information, the X-ray could be misinterpreted, leading one to think that stool in the cecum was actually stool in the rectum. When assessing a patient on a mechanical emptying regimen, you must ensure that the rectum and descending colon are clean. This could inadvertently cause you to strengthen a flush, thinking there is stool remaining in the rectum when in fact the colon is clean.

QUESTION 33.15

What does the contrast study in Figure 33.15 represent?

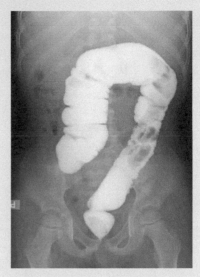

Figure 33.15 Contrast study question mark.

Answer: This contrast study looks a lot like a question mark, particularly if one could add a white dot at the bottom. Since you are becoming an expert in colorectal care, you might be asked to give some talks about the subject. Consider using this slide at the end of your talk when you want to elicit questions from the audience.

PART VII

MYTHS

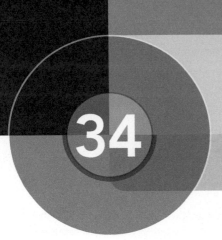

Colorectal surgical myths

34

JULIE M. CHOUEIKI

CASE STUDY 1

A 13-year-old male with a history of Hirschsprung disease is referred to your clinic. The patient has total colonic Hirschsprung disease (TCHD) with a transition in the terminal ileum. The patient did well in his first year of life after the creation of a diverting ileostomy in the newborn period. When he was about 1 year old, he underwent a colectomy and a straight endorectal pull-through. Pathology confirmed the original diagnosis of TCHD. One year after pull-through, the patient suffered from frequent episodes of enterocolitis, which required daily colonic irrigations, 3 episodes of intravenous fluid treatment for dehydration, and antibiotics.

Repeat pathology obtained at the age of 5 confirmed the presence of ganglion cells in the neorectum. The patient underwent an anal myomectomy in an attempt to treat continued episodes of enterocolitis.

QUESTION 34.1

What do you think of this procedure?

Answer: A myomectomy would not be recommended as it can permanently injure the sphincters. Instead, botulinum toxin is recommended as it is effective, can be repeated as necessary, and is the preferred alternative to a myomectomy.

The patient has daily soiling, both at night and during the day, that requires him to wear a sanitary napkin. He takes 6 mg of loperamide (Imodium) once daily. He is not on any fiber supplements. He is continent of urine but does have occasional accidents. He has not suffered from urinary tract infections and takes no urinary medications.

QUESTION 34.2

Do you believe there is any hope for fecal continence in this patient? What would you need to find out first about this patient?

Answer: You believe you can offer help to this patient. You choose to evaluate the integrity of the dentate line and whether the myectomy has compromised the sphincters. An anorectal manometry (AMAN) test while the patient is awake will help determine if the sphincters are weakened.

Prior to the examination under anesthesia (EUA), you obtain an AMAN under general anesthesia, as the patient is unable to tolerate the study awake due to generalized anxiety. The study reveals low anal sphincter pressure.

QUESTION 34.3

What does the EUA in Figure 34.1 reveal?

Answer: The EUA reveals that the dentate line is absent.

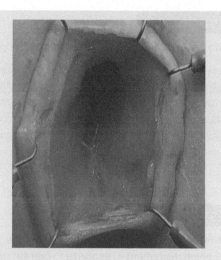

Figure 34.1 (See color insert.) EUA showing a last dentate line.

Myth: A patient with Hirschsprung disease cannot be continent without having an intact dentate line. This concept has been proposed, but we believe the issue is more complex. Perhaps adequate sphincters can overcome a missing dentate line.

QUESTION 34.4

What is the likely reason for the absence of the dentate line?

Answer: It is likely that the surgeon started their pull-through too low.

In addition to an absent dentate line, the sphincters are patulous but intact. The pull-through is not twisted and you do not find an obstructing cuff or anastomotic stricture. You are able to pass a size 20 Hegar dilator. The previous biopsy you reviewed showed ganglion cells. An X-ray was obtained for this patient.

QUESTION 34.5

What does the image in Figure 34.2 show?

Answer: Minimal to no formed stool is appreciated on this X-ray. Based on the AMAN, EUA findings, and the X-ray, you believe you can keep the patient socially continent of stool. The presence of intact sphincters, although patulous, along with the lack of a significant stricture,

twist, or cuff leads you to believe that you can bulk the stool and slow down its movement through the colon. Had the sphincters been further damaged, you would not be hopeful for social continence for this patient.

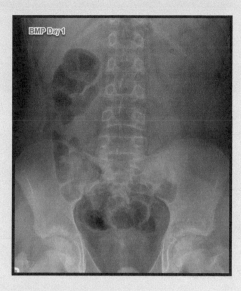

Figure 34.2 EUA TCHD patient.

QUESTION 34.6

What type of bowel management regimen would best support this goal?

Answer: You believe you can keep the neorectum area clean from stool in the evening to avoid soiling at night and bulk the stool during the day to prevent smears. During the day, the absent rectoanal inhibitory reflex (RAIR) plus voluntary sphincters should help keep the patient from soiling (helped by the bulked stool). At night, with external sphincters not in use, soiling is worse. You begin a week of a bowel management program (BMP) with adjusted regimens based on daily plain film X-rays to assess stool load. The starting regimen for BMP will consist of 6 mg of loperamide (Imodium) twice per day (BID), 3 grams of Nutrisource (guar gum) fiber BID (6 g daily total), and 1 suppository of bisacodyl to empty the neorectum before bed. Your rationale for utilizing the Imodium and fiber is to add bulk to the stool and prevent smears during the day, while the bisacodyl will serve as a stimulant laxative to facilitate the movement of the now-bulked stool at the appropriate time (Figure 34.3).

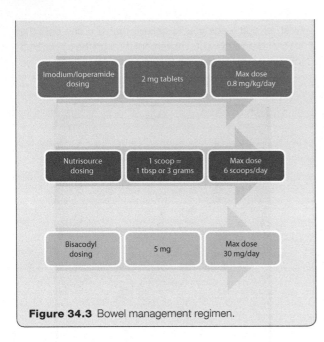

Figure 34.3 Bowel management regimen.

BMP DAY 3

QUESTION 34.7

What does the image in Figure 34.4 show?

Answer: The X-ray reveals minimal retained stool. Three days into the BMP week, the patient reports he is doing better. He reports 6–9 controlled bowel movements per day with no accidents during the day, but still has soiling every night in bed.

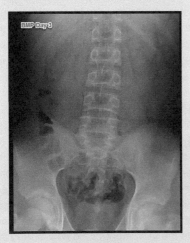

Figure 34.4 X-ray BMP Day 3.

QUESTION 34.8

Why do you suspect nighttime soiling is still happening?

Answer: You believe the patient needs more bulk to the stool. The patient reports increased sensation of "fullness" in the rectum when he has to have a bowel movement. He reports tolerating the medications with no discomfort. The patient has been able to do the bisacodyl suppository at night without difficulty.

QUESTION 34.9

What is your plan for day 3 of bowel management week, given the patient's response to current regimen, history, and X-ray (Figure 34.4)?

Answer: You plan to continue 6 mg of Imodium BID (AM and PM), increase the dose of Nutrisource to 6 grams BID to further bulk the stool and prevent smearing, and continue the suppository.

BMP DAY 5

QUESTION 34.10

What does the image in Figure 34.5 show?

Answer: Imaging shows small appreciable stool.

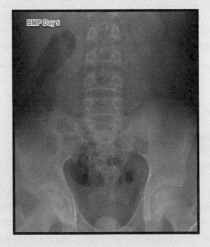

Figure 34.5 X-ray BMP Day 5.

QUESTION 34.11

What is your plan after day 5 of bowel management week, given the patient's response to the current regimen and X-ray (Figure 34.5)?

Answer: You choose to continue to increase the bulking agents to your regimen, specifically increasing the Imodium to 8 mg BID and continue dosing the Nutrisource at 3 g three times a day (TID). You also increase the stimulant bisacodyl to two suppositories, 30 minutes after dinner. Your goal is to increase the bulking and slow the movement of the stool while stimulating the colon to empty at the appropriate time.

BMP DAY 6

QUESTION 34.12

What does the image in Figure 34.6 show?

Answer: The imaging shows no appreciable stool or significant fecal material. At the completion of BMP week, the patient reported fewer accidents during the day, a few small smears, and multiple controlled stools per day during the day, yet still has an accident in his pull-up overnight.

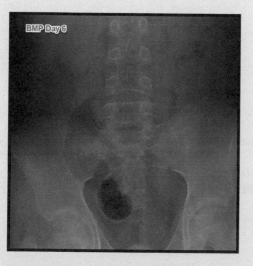

Figure 34.6 X-ray BMP Day 6.

QUESTION 34.13

What is your plan after day 6 of bowel management week, given the patient's response to current regimen (unchanged) and X-ray (Figure 34.6)?

Answer: You send the patient home with a plan to increase the dose of Imodium to 10 mg BID, increase Nutrisource to 9 grams twice per day, and continue with 2 bisacodyl suppositories, 30 minutes after dinner. You instruct the patient to follow up in one month.

QUESTION 34.14

The patient calls 10 days later and reports occasional smearing with nighttime incontinence. Do you make any adjustments to his medication regimen?

Answer: You elect to increase the Imodium to 12 mg BID and give the evening dose at bedtime to continue to attempt to slow down the patient's motility at night. You plan for a 1-month post–BMP week follow-up visit.

At 1 month you conduct a follow-up phone call with the patient. Outside images report mild stool density and no significant constipation. The current medication regimen for this patient 1 month after completion of the BMP week is Imodium 12 mg BID, Nutrisource 9 grams BID, and 2 bisacodyl suppositories after dinner. He is not on a specific diet plan, but eats mostly pasta, bread, and cheese. You recommend a constipating diet consisting of foods such as plain rice milk, applesauce, bananas, white and refined flour (bread, crackers, pasta, noodles, rice, peeled potatoes), and meats (baked, broiled, or grilled). Foods to be avoided include fresh vegetables, raw fruits, sugar (sweets and drinks such as sodas and juices), beans, fried foods, and butter.

He reports that his stooling status has improved. He is stooling at least 7–10 times per day and reports being continent during the day with only occasional smearing. He remains incontinent of stool overnight. His stool consistency is soft to loose. Of note, his mother states that they ran out of bisacodyl suppositories a couple of days ago and patient reports he feels his overnight stooling is less than it was when he was taking the suppositories.

What is your future plan for this patient as you have reached your goal of social (daytime) continence, with infrequent smearing and continued nighttime incontinence?

Answer: You advise the patient to avoid laxative foods and incorporate more constipating foods. You recommend stopping the bisacodyl suppositories, as the patient has stated they are ineffective. You advise changing the timing and dosage of Imodium 8 mg TID

and Nutrisource 6 grams TID. You recommend starting Levsin (hyoscyamine) ½ tablet BID. The Levsin will help to slow motility further. You request a report from the patient 1–2 weeks after the new regimen has been started and discuss slowly titrating up Levsin and possibly adding a small saline enema at night.

While you recognize you are fine-tuning the regimen to eliminate any nocturnal encopresis, the patient and family are overjoyed to have achieved daytime social fecal continence despite his diagnosis of TCHD and no dentate line.

KEY LEARNING POINTS

1. A nighttime enema can help avoid nighttime soiling.
2. What other options could have been utilized to slow down the stool (Figure 34.7)?
3. What recommendations would you make for a constipating diet?
   i. The constipating diet can be done in two phases. In phase 1, your child will strictly eat constipating foods to control the watery stools and help slow down the bowel. The second phase will begin 24 to 48 hours after your child has not had any accidents and involves slowly adding fats. During phase 2, you will want to add a new food (one at a time), every 2 to 3 days and closely watch to see if your child has an accident (Tables 34.1 and 34.2).

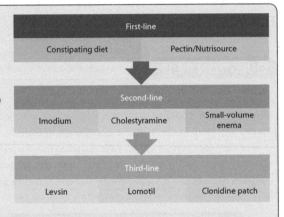

Figure 34.7 Hypermotility.

Table 34.1 Constipating diet phase 1

Food group	Food recommendations	Foods to avoid or limit
Milk	Plain rice milk	All others
Vegetables	None	If vegetables are eaten, make sure they are cooked and not raw
Fruits	Applesauce, apples (without skin), bananas	Avoid raw fruits
Starch, grains	White flour, refined flour	All others
	Bread, crackers, pasta and noodles, white rice, white potatoes (without skin), dry cereals	
Meat, seafood, legumes	Baked/broiled/grilled meats, poultry or fish, lean deli meats, eggs	Avoid beans
Fats, oils	Nonstick spray, nonfat butter spray	Limit butter, margarine, and oils No fried foods
Sweets	Sugar-free gelatin, popsicles, jelly, or syrup Rice-milk ice cream	All others
Beverages	Water, Gatorade, sugar-free Crystal Light, sugar-free Kool-Aid, Pedialyte	Avoid carbonated beverages, soda, juices, high-sugar drinks

Table 34.2 Constipating diet phase 2

Food group	Food recommendations	Foods to avoid
Milk	All milk products allowed, but limit to 500 mL total per day	Any milk or cheese products (such as ice cream) with nuts or seeds
Vegetables	Vegetable juice without pulp, vegetables that are well cooked	Raw vegetables
		Vegetables with seeds
	Green beans, spinach, pumpkin, eggplant, potatoes (without skin), asparagus, beets, carrots	
Fruits	Applesauce, apples (without skin), banana, melon, canned fruit, fruit juice (without pulp)	Fruit juice with pulp, canned pineapple, prunes, dried fruit, jam, marmalade
Starch, grains	Bread, crackers, cereals made from refined flours	Whole-grain or seeded breads
	Pasta or noodles made from white flours	Whole-grain pasta
	White rice, pretzels, white potatoes (without skin), dry cereal	Brown rice, oatmeal, bran cereal, whole-grain cereal
Meat, seafood, legumes	Meat, poultry, eggs, seafood	Beans
	Baked, broiled or grilled are preferred cooking methods	Fried or greasy meats, salami, cold cuts, hot dogs, meat substitutes
Fats, oils	All oils, margarine, butter, mayonnaise, salad dressings	Chunky peanut butter, nuts, seeds, coconut
Sweets	Jelly, Rice Dream frozen desserts, sugar, marshmallows, angel food cake	Anything containing nuts, coconut, whole-grains, dried fruits, or jams
Beverages	Water, Gatorade, sugar-free Crystal Light, sugar-free Kool-Aid, Pedialyte	Juice, regular soda, regular Kool-Aid, or powdered drinks
Miscellaneous	Salt, sugar, ground or flaked herbs and spices, vinegar, ketchup, mustard and soy sauce	Popcorn, pickles, horseradish, relish, jams, preserves

CASE STUDY 2

A 13-year-old male is referred to your center. The patient was adopted from China at the age of 7 with an unknown original anorectal malformation. There is a retracted left lower quadrant scar you believe is from a colostomy closure site.

QUESTION 34.16

Initially what type of malformation do you suspect?

Answer: You suspect the malformation was originally a rectourethral fistula due to the colostomy closure site scar.

The patient has 7 controlled bowel movements a day and experiences accidents or incontinence up to 4 days each week, averaging 3–6 accidents per week. He reports limited sensation with bowel movements, stating he, "can't feel it and it just comes out." He has no abdominal distention or pain. Previous interventions for this incontinence have included a constipating diet and inpatient disimpaction. He takes Imodium (loperamide) 1–2 mg daily. He is continent of urine and voids 5–6 times per day, with no history of urinary tract infections.

Previous testing has included a normal contrast enema with satisfactory spontaneous evacuation of contrast and stool. His lateral sacral ratio is normal (0.92) and he has no tethered cord.

The parents state their goal for their son is to be continent of stool and able to participate freely in the multiple sports activities he desires.

QUESTION 34.17

What do you believe is needed for a patient with this history to become continent of stool? Do you predict bowel control?

Answer: *Myth:* A patient with an anorectal malformation (ARM) and no rectum cannot be continent.

You recognize that this patient, despite his ARM and past surgical history, can become continent if there are adequate sphincter muscles present, pelvic proprioception, and if you can achieve a good bowel movement pattern (1–2 well-formed stools per day).

The main predictors of continence in the ARM patient include the type of original malformation and quality of spine and sacrum. In this patient, we do not know the original malformation but he has a normal spine and sacrum (refer to the figure "ARM Index" in the color insert).

QUESTION 34.18

What would your evaluation include?

Answer: You plan for an exam under anesthesia (EUA), a contrast enema via the rectum, a pelvic ultrasound, a kidney ultrasound and a bowel management program (BMP). BMP will include 1 week of intense bowel management with serial X-rays and medication regimen changes as needed throughout the week.

Your EUA is completed and you find a well-centered anus surrounded by muscle complex having good contraction with stimulation. You are able to pass a size 18 Hegar dilator. There is no anal stricture present or rectal prolapse. The kidney ultrasound shows bilateral hydronephrosis, right greater than left; normal sonographic appearance; and the renal parenchyma without mass, cyst, or scar. There is moderate-to-large-volume post-void residual. The contrast enema via the rectum reveals a well-formed sacrum, normal caliber colon with redundant transverse colon. The presacral space is normal (see Figure 34.8).

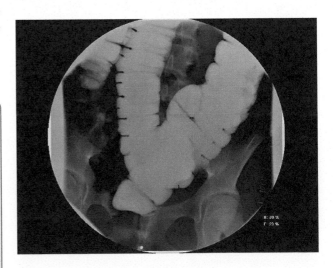

Figure 34.8 Contrast enema findings.

QUESTION 34.19

What does this tell you?

Answer: He has good anatomy and evidence of a well-done repair, except for the fact that the rectum was unfortunately discarded. It is likely that he originally underwent an abdominoperineal pull-through procedure. You can see haustrations in the pelvis, which means the sigmoid was pulled through.

The cecum is normally rotated into the right lower quadrant. No focal stricture or segmental dilation is present. The anal opening appears properly located. The colon is devoid of stool, with the patient evacuating a large majority of the introduced contrast.

QUESTION 34.20

Are you hopeful based on the findings that you can achieve social continence for this patient?

Answer: You believe that based on the continence predictors of type of **a**norectal malformation (low) and quality of **s**pine and **s**acrum (normal), you have good potential for bowel control (mnemonic A.S.S). Based on these findings you begin bowel management bootcamp to achieve social continence.

QUESTION 34.21

What medication regimen would you begin with for this patient?

Answer: You begin BMP day 1 with rectal enemas 400 mL saline, 20 mL glycerin, Imodium 1 mg PO BID, and Nutrisource 3 g TID (9 g). You start the patient on a constipating diet, as you predict hypermotility. Your goal is to mechanically empty the colon for 24 hours, remain accident free, and have no voluntary bowel managements aside from the enema. The glycerin serves as a stimulant to the bowel while the Imodium will increase bulk to the stool and slow the colon down between flushes.

BMP DAY 4

QUESTION 34.22

What does the X-ray in Figure 34.9 show you?

Answer: The X-ray shows minimal retained stool within the ascending colon and no appreciable stool in transverse, descending, sigmoid colons, or neorectum. The patient returns to clinic on day 4 of BMP and his parents report that the medication regimen was given as ordered. He is tolerating rectal enemas but has intermittent cramping throughout the day. The patient experienced 5 accidents that started after 9 pm, or 12 hours after the enema. Today, he had the enema and sat for 1 hour followed by a yellow liquid stool with some mushy stool 40 minutes later. He reports that 10 minutes after starting breakfast he could not make it to the bathroom. He continues to have difficulty feeling the stool, more so when it is liquid. The patient and his parents report that they have tried many combinations over the years with Imodium and fiber. His mother reports that the patient has tried as much as 4–5 mg of Imodium per day and it has not slowed down his stool frequency.

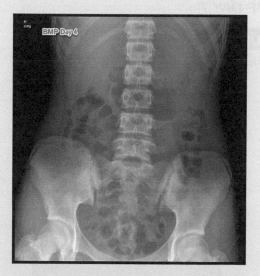

Figure 34.9 X-ray BMP Day 4.

QUESTION 34.23

What changes, if any, should be made to his medication regimen based on the radiological findings and the patient's report?

Answer: As the patient is reporting intermittent cramping throughout the day and night, with the knowledge that he has no rectum, and as evidenced by pronounced haustra, we should expect significant hypermotility. You believe his clean X-ray of stool is due to being overstimulated. You make the following medication regimen changes: decrease the enema to 400 mL of saline plus 10 mL of glycerin. You increase the bulk of his stools with an increase of the Nutrisource 2 tbsp (6 g) in the morning, 2 tbsp (6 g) in the afternoon and 1 tbsp (3 g) in the evening. You increase the Imodium to 2 mg PO BID to slow him down between the enemas. The patient is scheduled to meet with the dietician as well to discuss a constipating diet.

BMP DAY 6

Patient reports cramping and his flush is decreased to 400 mL of saline and 5 mL of glycerin.

BMP DAY 7

QUESTION 34.24

What does the X-ray in Figure 34.10 show you?

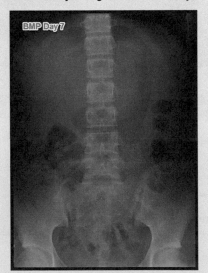

Figure 34.10 X-ray BMP Day 7.

Answer: The patient's X-ray shows stool within the ascending colon. There is otherwise no appreciable stool in the transverse, descending, or sigmoid colon. On day 7 BMP the patient reports that he has not experienced any accidents for 2 days. You keep his bowel regimen as prescribed for him to return home and plan for 1-month, 3-month, and 1-year follow-up visits.

QUESTION 34.25

What future surgical procedure might improve his quality of life if enemas are to be continued long term for this patient?

Answer: The possibility of a Malone is introduced to the family for future consideration.

A 1-month follow-up phone call is conducted. The mother reports that the patient has adjusted the flush to 350 mL of saline and 20 mL of glycerin. He continues with Imodium 2 mg TID and Nutrisource 6 g TID. He has been continent with this regimen and no accidents. A recent X-ray showed no appreciable stool. You advise the patient to transition to evening rectal enemas by doing two flushes one day and then resuming in the evening. You advise that he may have an additional Imodium dose on the day of transition. His parents report that patient is currently experiencing social continence and that it is, "life changing."

SUGGESTED READING

Lane, V. I., Skerrit, C., Wood, R. et al. 2016. A standardized approach for the assessment and treatment of internationally adopted children with a previously repaired anorectal malformation (ARM). *Journal of Pediatric Surgery*, 51, 1864–1870.

Levitt, M. A., Dickie, B., & Pena, A. 2010. Evaluation and treatment of the patient with Hirschsprung's disease who is not doing well after a pull-through procedure. *Seminars in Pediatric Surgery*, 19(2), 146–153.

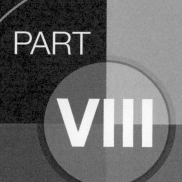

PART

VIII

MEDICATION
PROTOCOLS

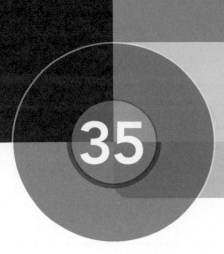

Medication protocols

MEGHAN FISHER AND ONNALISA NASH

HYPOMOTILITY

LAXATIVES: SENNA

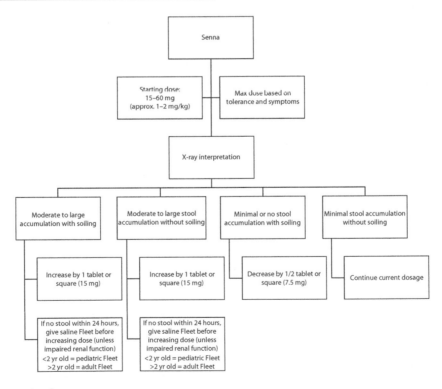

Figure 35.1 Senna protocol.

- Start fiber (Figure 35.2) if stool is loose on senna regimen (Figure 35.1).
- If patient is intolerant to senna, stop senna and switch to bisacodyl (Figure 35.3).

FIBER (WITH LAXATIVES)

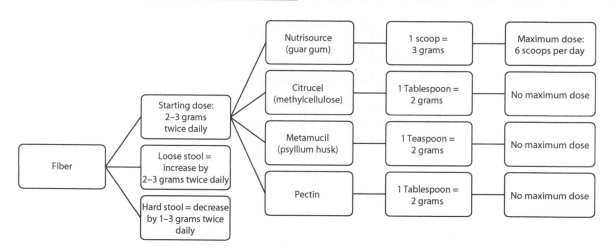

Figure 35.2 Fiber protocol.

LAXATIVES: BISACODYL

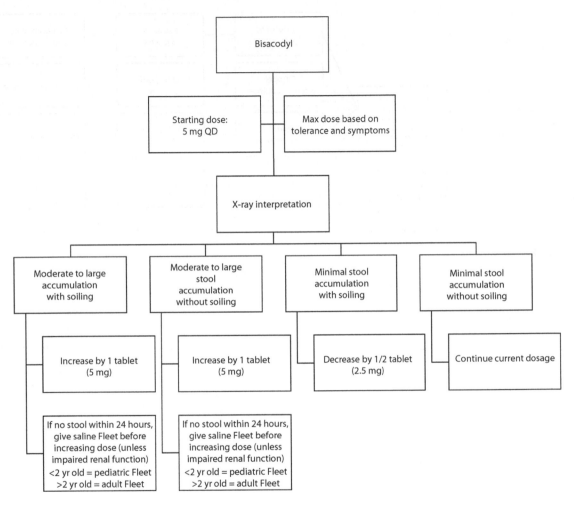

Figure 35.3 Oral bisacodyl protocol.

- Start fiber if stool is loose on bisacodyl regimen.

FLUSHES: SALINE AND GLYCERIN

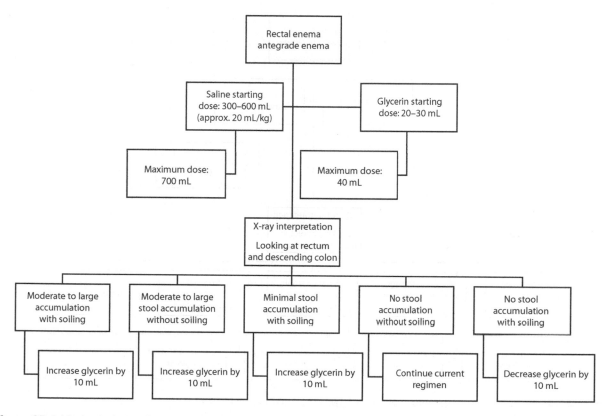

Figure 35.4 Mechanical emptying protocol with saline and glycerin.

- Continue on pathway (Figure 35.4) until glycerin is maximized or patient is unable to tolerate stimulant. Significant side effects may include severe cramping, nausea, vomiting, etc.
- Consider adding Castile soap (Figure 35.5) to current regimen or using Castile soap as primary stimulant if tolerance is an issue.

FLUSHES: SALINE, GLYCERIN, AND CASTILE

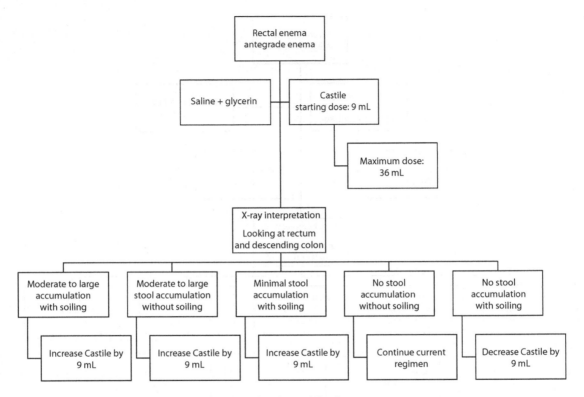

Figure 35.5 Mechanical emptying protocol with saline, glycerin, and Castile soap.

FLUSH: BISACODYL

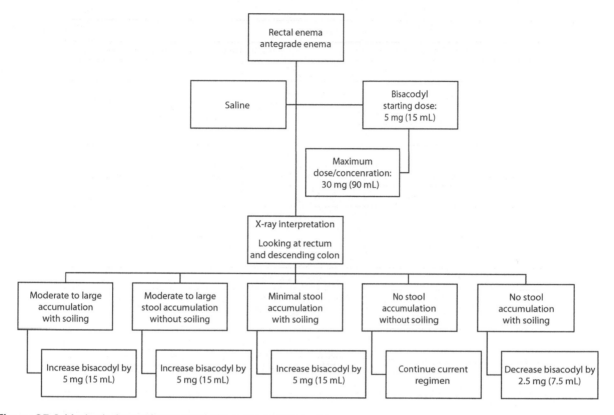

Figure 35.6 Mechanical emptying protocol with saline and bisacodyl.

- If patient is intolerant or not responding to max dose of glycerin and/or Castile, switch stimulant to bisacodyl enema liquid (Figure 35.6). Use with caution in patients with anorectal malformation (ARM).

HYPERMOTILITY

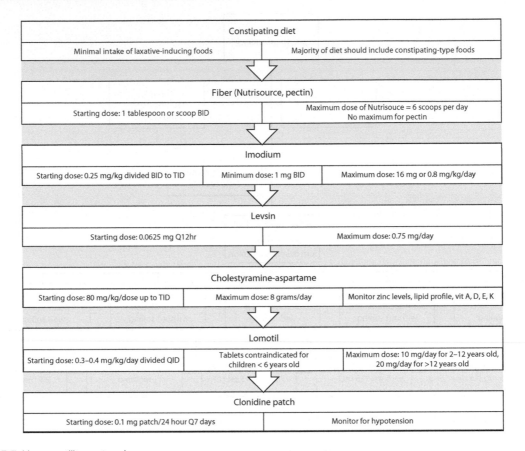

Constipating diet		
Minimal intake of laxative-inducing foods		Majority of diet should include constipating-type foods

Fiber (Nutrisource, pectin)		
Starting dose: 1 tablespoon or scoop BID		Maximum dose of Nutrisouce = 6 scoops per day No maximum for pectin

Imodium		
Starting dose: 0.25 mg/kg divided BID to TID	Minimum dose: 1 mg BID	Maximum dose: 16 mg or 0.8 mg/kg/day

Levsin	
Starting dose: 0.0625 mg Q12hr	Maximum dose: 0.75 mg/day

Cholestyramine-aspartame		
Starting dose: 80 mg/kg/dose up to TID	Maximum dose: 8 grams/day	Monitor zinc levels, lipid profile, vit A, D, E, K

Lomotil		
Starting dose: 0.3–0.4 mg/kg/day divided QID	Tablets contraindicated for children < 6 years old	Maximum dose: 10 mg/day for 2–12 years old, 20 mg/day for >12 years old

Clonidine patch	
Starting dose: 0.1 mg patch/24 hour Q7 days	Monitor for hypotension

Figure 35.7 Hypermotility protocol.

Continue medication until the maximum dose is reached. Once the maximum dose is reached, add in the next medication. Continue adding medications to regimen until desired stool consistency and frequency are obtained (Figure 35.7).

Flushes:

- Consider small-volume enemas for nighttime soiling and/or severe perineal breakdown
- 100–200 mL saline before bed or twice daily
- Continue hypermotile medications to slow down stool between flushes

Ileostomy:

- Consider for ongoing soiling, severe perineal breakdown, diminished quality of life, and failure to thrive

OTHER CONSIDERATIONS

1. Add fiber to a flush regimen if the patient is soiling with a clean X-ray and lower dose of stimulant is not effective.
2. Dietary habits and recent changes. Encourage the family to keep a food diary.
3. Hardened stool with flush:
   A. Add 1 capful of polyethylene glycol 3350 (MiraLAX) 6–8 hours prior to flush, taken orally
4. Right colon accumulation with Malone:
   A. Separate bisacodyl from flush by administering bisacodyl alone first, follow with saline flush
   B. Lay on right side during flush
   C. Add 1–2 capfuls of polyethylene glycol 3350 (MiraLAX) 30–60 minutes prior to flush directly into Malone
   D. Administer sodium phosphate enema (Fleet) (unless impaired renal function) 30 minutes prior to flush directly into Malone
      i. Check renal labs every 3–6 months
5. Maximum dose of all stimulants without clearance on X-ray
   A. Use polyethylene glycol 3350 and electrolytes (GoLYTELY) as base of flush instead of saline
6. Increasing volume of flush if only rectum and/or distal descending clean
7. Decreasing volume of flush if you visualize stool clearance past the splenic flexure
8. Failure of medical management
   A. Anorectal malformation
      i. Malone
   B. Hirschsprung disease
      i. Malone
      ii. Botulinum toxin
   C. Spinal anomaly
      i. Malone
   D. Functional constipation
      i. Anorectal manometry (AMAN)
         – Withholding—Botulinum toxin
         – Absent rectoanal inhibitory reflex (RAIR)—rectal biopsy to rule out Hirschsprung disease
      ii. Colonic manometry (CMAN)
         – Segmental dysmotility—Malone
            A. If Malone is successful, retry laxatives in 6 months to 1 year
            B. If Malone is unsuccessful, retest colon with CMAN
               i. If dysmotile segment found, colonic resection
         – Normal—Malone
            A. Laxative trial in 6 months to 1 year

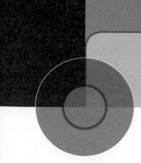

Index

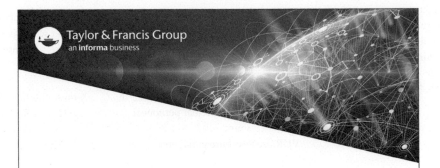